Global Health in the Global North

This book investigates how health interventions are imagined into being in high-income countries, drawing on over seven years of fieldwork in the self-described "global health capital" Atlanta to consider the role of storytelling in the construction of global health futures.

The volume highlights the ways in which scientific storytelling is critical to our understanding of how global health futures are constructed. The book examines three value types—epistemic, ethical, and economic—central to contemporary global health and three linguistic and communicative phenomena—multimodal poetics, emplotment, and discursive circulation—significant to the constitution of these values through storytelling. In spotlighting the Atlanta metropolitan region, home to a number of prominent organizations and figures in the development of global health, the book showcases deeper insights into the future-oriented and techno-optimistic stories global health professionals tell each other, funders, and the public. Black builds on these discussions to suggest ways forward for these stories to be improved to foster greater equity and decolonization and reimagine the future of global health.

This book will be of interest to students and scholars in linguistic anthropology, medical anthropology, global health, and health humanities.

Steven P. Black is Professor of Anthropology at Georgia State University, USA.

Routledge Studies in Health Humanities

The Languages of COVID-19
Translational and Multilingual Perspectives on Global Healthcare
Edited by Piotr Blumczynski and Steven Wilson

The Social, Aesthetic, and Medical Implications of Performing Shame
Interdisciplinary Approaches
Marlene Goldman

Pandemic Health and Fitness
Sabina M. Perrino and Joshua O. Reno

Planetary Health Humanities and Pandemics
Edited by Heike Härting and Heather Meek

Language, Pharmacy and Society
The Sounds of Local Knowledges and the Linguistic Logistics of Science
Milton Fernando Gonzalez Rodriguez

Global Health in the Global North
Techno-Optimism and the Value of Storytelling for the Future of Health Equity
Steven P. Black

For more information about this series, please visit: https://www.routledge.com/Routledge-Studies-Health-Humanities/book-series/RSH

Global Health in the Global North

Techno-Optimism and the Value of Storytelling for the Future of Health Equity

Steven P. Black

Routledge
Taylor & Francis Group
NEW YORK AND LONDON

First published 2025
by Routledge
605 Third Avenue, New York, NY 10158

and by Routledge
4 Park Square, Milton Park, Abingdon, Oxon, OX14 4RN

Routledge is an imprint of the Taylor & Francis Group, an informa business

ISBN: 9781032910284 (hbk)
ISBN: 9781032910307 (pbk)
ISBN: 9781003561019 (ebk)

DOI: 10.4324/9781003561019

Typeset in Sabon
by codeMantra

In what those who know me well would describe as typical fashion, it took me a long time to realize that this project held personal and familial significance for me. When it comes to career, my narrative has long been that in college I turned away from the family business—that business being physics. My maternal grandfather was a physicist, as was my maternal uncle, one of my maternal cousins, and my older brother. And math and science always came naturally to me, so I suppose it would not have been unexpected for me to become a physicist. Indeed, as a freshman at UCLA I enrolled in "Chemistry for Physical Science Majors," fully intending to follow that path. But I was also a jazz saxophonist with a passion for music, so I decided to concurrently enroll in an ethnomusicology course, "Music and Culture of the Near East and Africa." From my youthful perspective, the juxtaposition of these two courses could not have made things clearer. The ethnomusicology class was vibrant, exciting, and interesting. The chemistry course was dry and dull (which was probably actually more of an indication of the professor than the subject). Within a week, I had dropped the chemistry course. Soon after I was a double-major in anthropology and ethnomusicology, and the rest is history.

As I write this, though, I am reminded that there is a whole other cast of characters—another part of my family—that are elided from the plot of this story. This includes educators (my mother and sister), a social worker (my paternal aunt), and a nurse (my paternal grandmother). Even my maternal grandfather (the physicist) primarily studied medical physics, contributing to the development of X-ray and MRI technologies. This includes my father and paternal grandfather. Before retiring, my father was a lawyer. He worked for the California Department of Mental Health for almost the entirety of his career. And my paternal grandfather worked for the US Department of Public Health as an environmental engineer (his work contributed to the founding of the Environmental Protection Agency). Growing up, I heard my father talk about the dynamics of the California public health system in the wake of Ronald Reagan's governorship. After I moved to Los Angeles to attend UCLA, my paternal grandfather liked to remind me that I could contract malaria there even though it was not as common as it once was (a fun fact to share). I later learned that one of his signature contributions to the field of waste management was a careful study of landfills. He calculated the precise amount of soil that had to be spread over a landfill to prevent the breeding of flies and other problematic disease-spreading insects.

So I got my first exposure to some of the key themes of this book, such as the impacts of neoliberal governance on health care and the significance of data-driven approaches for public health, around the dinner table and at family gatherings during my youth. So I would like to dedicate this book to all my extended family, including my maternal grandmother (not yet mentioned), who never completed a college degree but was nonetheless the one to introduce me to that deeply ambivalent phrase, "publish or perish!"

Contents

Figures

Excerpts

Acknowledgments

This book has been a long time in the making, so I may have forgotten some of the contributions of others along the way, but I am hopeful that I have not left anyone out of these acknowledgments. First and foremost, I would like to thank my spouse: intrepid linguistic anthropologist Elizabeth Falconi. She has shaped this book in a myriad of ways, always generously ready to listen to and provide feedback on my ideas whenever I get stuck or discouraged, caring for our children when I traveled to Costa Rica each summer for several years for this project, and working tirelessly with me to make a life for our family in Decatur, Georgia (the setting for much of the book).

I would like to thank the individuals who were interviewed for this project for their generosity and time—including several friends and acquaintances—who are referred to using pseudonyms to protect confidentiality. And I would like to acknowledge David Ross of the Taskforce for Global Health for meeting with me and encouraging me in this work. I would like to express gratitude to my friend Garrett Assay, who is an economist and public health specialist, for always being open to having informal conversations about new ideas and observations that I came up with during the course of the project. And thanks to Charles Briggs for conversations and suggestions about which publishers to reach out to with the proposal for this interdisciplinary text.

I would also like to thank Carlos Faerron Guzmán, who is a friend, global health scholar, and research/teaching collaborator, for reading and providing feedback on Chapter 1 and—along with Carolina Bolaños Palmieri (thank you Caro!)—for collaborating in the design and implementation of a global health study abroad program and a planetary health research project. And thank you to Alessandro Duranti in his role as editor for a book series, and to other editors of that book series, for reading and providing very helpful feedback on a previous draft of the book.

I also received valuable feedback while presenting various parts of this project at several conferences and seminars. This included the University of California, Los Angeles Center for Language, Interaction, and Culture (thank you for the invitation to present and for providing significant early feedback on the project); a 2021 panel I participated in (organized by Martha Lincoln) for the Society for Social Studies of Science Annual meeting; a panel I organized for the 2022 *American Anthropological Association meeting* on "Language and Public/ Global Health" (thank you to fellow presenters Ashlee Dauphinais Civitello and Paja Faudree and discussant Martha Lincoln); a double panel I co-organized with Kathryn Graber on value and semiotics for the 2023 American Anthropological Association meeting in Toronto (thank you to Kathryn and fellow presenters Lynda Chubak, Sherina Feliciano-Santos, Mathias Levi Toft Kristiansen, Motserrat Perez Castro Perez, Alessandra Rosen, Matt Schneider, Shalini Shankar, Daniel Souleles, and discussants Josh Reno and Jillian Cavanaugh). Also, thank you to Denise Davidson and other attendees of the Georgia State University's Humanities Research Center 2023 faculty fellows seminar for feedback on Chapter 2. And thank you to Andrew Buskell and Helen Curry, organizers of the Georgia Institute of Technology's Metro Atlanta Science Studies Seminar, and attendees of the seminar (especially Cindy Kaiying Lin), for feedback on Chapter 5.

Limited funding for this project was provided by Georgia State University, in the form of a Humanities Research Center Maymester Fellowship and a Research Intensive Semester (RISe) award (what used to be called sabbaticals, but now we are required to apply for them and continue doing service work during the semester).

1 Introduction

Dear reader,

It feels a little bit strange to publish a book on "global health equity" at a time when the concept of equity and the fields of public and global health themselves are under political attack in the US. Those whose livelihoods and life's work are threatened may not currently have the time nor the inclination to rethink the role of techno-optimism in the field as they are scrambling to find any funding at all to continue their efforts to save the lives of some of the world's most marginalized people. At the same time, though, maintaining an intellectual forum to reconsider concepts such as health equity, North-South relations, and the social determinants of health is more relevant than ever—if not for the current struggles then for a possible future in which global and public health professionals may once more be free to design and plan health interventions. And this book is, after all, about imagining values into being, so I invite readers to look toward the future with me and to critically and creatively envision what global health in the global North could and should be like in the years to come.

***

In Decatur, Georgia (a city in the metropolitan Atlanta area with about 24,000 residents) on a chilly but sunny January morning in 2019, I am walking my five-year-old daughter to her public elementary school with my three-year-old son in tow in a stroller. The many trees lining the quiet two-lane roads are bare of leaves. While I do not spot any parents in uniform on this morning, we often do see commissioned corps members of the Centers for Disease Control and Prevention (CDC)—whose offices are located less than two miles away—in full military dress. CDC, alongside Emory University (a public and global health education powerhouse), are important employers in the area. Indeed, as one Decatur-based journalist said, "You can't throw a rock without hitting a Ph.D. around here" (Ellis and O'Donnell 2020).[1] And Decatur is located in metropolitan Atlanta, which is a self-described "global health capital."[2]

DOI: 10.4324/9781003561019-1

Like many of my public and global health neighbors, my spouse and I are transplants with advanced degrees who moved to the Atlanta area for employment. And like many, we chose to live in the city of Decatur because we valued its walkability, relative diversity, and strong public school system, along with its proximity to our places of employment and affordability for those on government salaries. In other words, we moved here with a clear understanding of the value of the city in terms of what public health calls the social determinants of health—"the conditions in which people are born, grow, work, live, and age, and the wider set of forces and systems shaping the conditions of daily life."[3]

After saying goodbye to my daughter, my son and I begin the trek home, walking past craftsman bungalows interspersed with newer "tear down" replacement two-story homes towering over them (a sign of the ongoing gentrification of the neighborhood). We run into an acquaintance who lives down the street. She is also walking back to her house after dropping off her kids at school. Exchanging greetings, I ask, "do I remember correctly that you work in global health?" She replies yes. I explain that I am doing a project studying global health, specifically examining global health discourses (a fairly vague and amorphous idea) and we start to talk as we walk.

I mention to her that many of the people I've met who work in Atlanta and work in global health seem to be a tight-knit group. I joke that they always seem to be meeting with Jim Kim (a former head of the World Bank who studied anthropology) and Paul Farmer (a physician/anthropologist who was world renowned before his death in 2022 for his global health work and his non-profit organization [NPO] Partners in Health).[4] My neighbor laughs, then confirms, "I've totally met Jim Kim and Paul Farmer multiple times!"

Our playful exchange points toward something that many do not realize. Most people think of global health as something that happens far away in the global South—that is, in low-income settings in places like Africa, North America south of the Río Grande river, South America, and Asia. And indeed, this is true. But many global health interventions are actually planned in the global North—in high-income places like Atlanta, Seattle (home to the Bill and Melinda Gates Foundation), Washington, DC, New York (home to the Rockefeller Foundation), and Geneva, Switzerland (home to the United Nations (UN) and World Health Organization) (see Brada 2011 on space and the inequities of global health).[5] In fact, a recent commentary argues, "Global health remains much too centred on individuals and agencies in high-income countries," and calls for global health decision-making to shift to low- and middle-income countries (Abimbola and Pai 2020: 1627).

Much scholarship that critically examines the field of global health focuses on the experience of those in the global South and is based on fieldwork conducted there (e.g., Hall-Clifford 2024; Keshavjee 2014). But what of those high-income spaces where priorities are often set and many interventions are crafted? I began my ethnographic research project in 2016 in the Atlanta metropolitan area hoping to address this dearth by focusing on global health professionals in the global North. However, I quickly ran into a problem. Despite several meetings with very polite and collegial leaders of global health organizations who agreed to share my emails to recruit interviewees, no one would consent to allow me to conduct participant observation embedded within their organization. Such challenges in accessing research sites and participants are a common issue for scholars who are "studying up"—doing research with people in positions of power and authority (Gusterson 1997; more on this below; Souleles 2018). It seemed like some of these leaders simply could not conceptualize the possibility that an anthropologist would want to do fieldwork in a global health organization home office. To many, anthropologists are social scientists whose expertise is in the "culture" of people far away (often in low-income settings) and our value to global health is primarily our ability to address "cultural barriers" to successful health interventions. Regardless of the reason, though, NPO leaders did not want me hanging out in their offices on a day-to-day basis, observing and documenting the mundane everyday world of global health.

On that chilly January morning in 2019 as I am walking alongside my neighbor, I mention this challenge of my research. Maybe one reason global health professionals do not want me to conduct participant observation at their offices, I suggest, is that they do not think there is much to observe, because they are often sitting in front of a computer. In response, she tells me that when she worked for the CDC Foundation (an NPO associated with CDC), an older colleague told her that the unsung hero of the Smallpox Eradication Program (in the 1960s and 1970s) was a CDC employee who never traveled (discussed in Chapter 2). He was the one with the phone, the maps, and the data, who sat at his desk, got people supplies, and dealt with logistical issues when they happened.

This brief story, retold by my neighbor (in other words, a circulating story), indicates that many Atlanta-based global health professionals are the global health equivalent of white-collar workers. They are middle to upper management in the world of global health. However, it is also true that many have previous experience working as physicians and epidemiologists in global health interventions in low-income and middle-income countries. In fact, to access certain promotions at CDC one must do a multi-year stint abroad (as I write this, one of our neighbors is currently in Indonesia for precisely this reason). After gaining that experience, though, a substantial number of people shift to jobs that are based in Atlanta (perhaps with moderate work travel to intervention sites) and spend much of the rest of their careers in Atlanta and other global health cities of the global North planning out the interventions that happen abroad. This book is about the stories that these global health professionals tell as they fundraise, plan, and organize—about the ethical, economic, and epistemic values that are (re)constituted through their stories, about how and why they tell the kinds of stories that they do, what sorts of futures are imagined through these stories, and, finally, how different futures can be imagined with an eye to increasing health equity.

Overview

In many ways, my own career trajectory as an anthropologist has been similar to that of my global health colleagues, starting abroad in the global South and now doing work closer to home. I first conducted research abroad in 2008, completing nine months of fieldwork in South Africa and working closely with a Zulu gospel choir that was an HIV support group, an AIDS activist organization, and a performance troupe. Research participants for that project were recipients of aid, targets of global health interventions, and activists at home and abroad. One of my foci in South Africa was the ethics of peripheral participation in global health organizations and the overlap and (sometimes) conflict with research participants' ethical frameworks at home. Among other things, I learned that the patient-activists with whom I worked had benefited a great deal through their involvement with NPOs and multilateral agencies. However, they also felt excluded and, in some ways, exploited. In particular, they felt that their images and personal/organizational histories were being used to craft a hopeful story about global health success in combating HIV/AIDS. That story circulated globally to audiences in high-income countries like the United States and Great Britain, generating donations for NPOs. But these donations did not directly benefit the research participants whose stories were being told, in contrast to doctors, counselors, and other health professionals. This matches other research findings that critique the power dynamics at play in global health interventions (e.g., Benton 2015; Brada 2017, Büyüm et al. 2020; Crane 2013).

Still, I had met enough global health professionals to understand that many were working tirelessly on projects to which they had devoted their lives, believing them valuable (especially in the epistemic and ethical sense). I wanted to understand their roles and perspectives in greater detail, leading me to begin the Global Health Discourses Project.[6] This would evolve to include my collaboration with Costa Rican academics who trained American global health students (including the development of our own global health/anthropology study abroad course), analysis of publicly available online content associated with global health, and fieldwork in the Atlanta area.

Though I started the Global Health Discourses Project with a focus on ethics, I soon realized that I could not fully understand how ethical frameworks were being deployed without also examining the economic imperatives and scientific perspectives that were intertwined with the ethics of global health. This trichotomy—of ethics, economics, and epistemology—led me to questions about value and storytelling.

In this book, I describe what I have learned by studying how global health operates in the global North—specifically, how the interventions that take place in low-income and middle-income countries get imagined into being through storytelling in high-income settings. While this may seem less significant than the very important work being done in low-income and middle-income countries, my experience—alongside growing calls to "decolonize" global health, in part by taking some of the power of the field away from high-income NPOs—suggests that the work of secular global health NPOs in high-income settings deserves further scrutiny. Through this book, I hope to contribute not only to anthropological theory but also to global health itself, providing some suggestions for how the stories global health professionals tell might be altered in ways to better align with their own stated interest in promoting equity.

Techno-Optimism as Scientific Discourse, Story, and Value System

Global health professionals in high-income settings tell stories about diseases, cures, and interventions. They do so in planning sessions, grant applications, public symposia, yearly reports, and a host of other contexts. These stories tend to be optimistic, technology-focused, and universalizing in nature. They also tend to deploy racialized affect (Berg and Ramos-Zayas 2015) in ways that reinforce existing inequities. Epidemiologists, doctors, and others immersed in the culture of science may dismiss analysis of such global health stories as not part of "the science" itself.[7] However, these stories do shape the concerns, goals, and interventions of the field, and so they are indeed extremely relevant. To say that scientists tell stories is not to question the veracity of the facts underlying their narratives, but rather to recognize the role of poetics, verbal art, and performance in the collaborative construction of all meaning, including the construction of value systems in the social contexts in which science is embedded.

In many scientific contexts—public and global health included—dominant perspectives often coalesce around techno-optimism. Broadly, techno-optimism is the idea and/or feeling that complex problems can be solved with simple novel technological solutions (Avle et al. 2020). While optimism is oriented toward the future, it also shapes actions in the present: "the subject leans toward promises contained within the present moment of the encounter with her object" (Berlant 2011: 24). Optimism is a core orientation in many global health contexts (Closser 2012). This includes but is not limited to neoliberal optimism, in which persons remain "confident in markets, despite the compromises they face in its 'broken marketplace'" (Mei 2017: 391) (see also Keshavjee 2014).

And neoliberalism is itself rooted in post-World War II prosperity and a belief that "human well-being can best be advanced by liberating individual entrepreneurial freedoms and skills within an institutional framework characterized by strong private property rights, free markets, and free trade" (Harvey 2005: 2; see also Ortner 2016). One key aspect of this post-World War II optimism is a widespread confidence in the ability of science and technology to solve human problems. This idea has shaped cultural understandings of science across a range of disciplines, perhaps none more so than global health.

This book is not a critique of technological fixes, per se. Technological fixes can be wonderful and contribute to the real improvement of the health of humans and the planet. However, problems occur when technological fixes are touted as the only solutions, when funding for and attention to underlying structural (socioeconomic, historical) conditions are neglected, and when solutions for the global South are narrated into being in global North settings without the expertise and meaningful partnership of those from the South.

In this book, I interweave three key theoretical frameworks to understand techno-optimism in global health: (1) a critical medical anthropology approach to the study of scientific discourses, (2) an expansive linguistic anthropology perspective on storytelling and narrative, and (3) a cultural and linguistic anthropology viewpoint on values and value systems. The idea of combining such theories from linguistic and medical anthropology is fairly unusual but not unprecedented, and in fact a vibrant group of scholars has recently been working to create a novel body of literature at the nexus of the two subfields (Briggs and Faudree 2016; Arnold et al. Forthcoming). Charles L. Briggs (2020) explains this approach:

> Imagine you have a deck of cards. It has four suits, designated "language," "communication," "medicine," and "care." You throw them up into the air. As if by magic, they are transformed before landing, not just mixing cards from different suits but destabilizing their very categorical distinctions and distinctive markings, thereby challenging players to rethink the game entirely.
>
> (563)

This sort of destabilization of categorical distinctions is one of my goals in writing this book. In global health in the global North, language and medicine are not just juxtaposed but rather are co-constitutive (see Briggs 2021:

290; Briggs and Mantini-Briggs 2016). Below, I provide a brief introduction to the three key theoretical frameworks I have chosen for this task.

A Measured Critique of Scientific Discourse

In 2018, the *New York Times Magazine* published an article about the philosopher Bruno Latour and the field of Science and Technology Studies (STS). This article would prove to be remarkably incisive in hindsight in the later context of the erosion of public trust in health interventions that occurred during the COVID-19 pandemic. The topic of the article was Latour's defense of science. This was newsworthy because, among other interests, Latour was known for his early work on "the social construction of scientific facts" (Latour and Woolgar 1987 [1979]). His scholarship contributed to the development of social constructivism, a perspective that—when taken to its logical extreme, or, some would say, reduced to absurdity—would seem to deny the existence of facts or reality. Indeed, the *NYT Magazine* article recounts a story in which a well-known physicist, "who was under the impression that Latour and his STS colleagues thought that 'the laws of physics are mere social conventions,' invited them to jump out the window of his 21st-floor apartment" (Kofman 2018). Latour did not jump.

Latour explains his early approach to STS: "I think we were so happy to develop all this critique because we were so *sure* of the authority of science... and that the authority of science would be shared because there was a common world" (Kofman 2018). To this, anthropologist and STS pioneer Donna Haraway adds that public understandings of science have changed since the 1990s, and critical STS scholarship must now support scientific endeavors "without closing down the fact that science is a set of situated practices and not capital-S science." In other words, science is a human activity and, as such, is inherently a part of human cultural practices. This is particularly true of scientific medicine, where science must account for human behavior, and especially so in public health, where the science/human behavior nexus meets socioeconomic structure and cultural/political context. And yet there are, for all intents and purposes, still facts. Finding a balance between acknowledgment of the epistemic authority of science and recognition of its culturally situated nature is particularly delicate now, after a pandemic in which denials and perversions of science fueled political movements while simultaneously filling graveyards, and with an incoming federal administration that has so far and in the past been hostile to expertise in the field of public health.

I offer this book on global health storytelling in the spirit of Haraway's entreaty and Latour's comments. Relatively few scholars have linked the study of storytelling and narrative with the critical examination of science (but see Ochs, Gonzales, and Jacoby 1996; Briggs and Mantini-Briggs 2003, 2016).[8] Yet analysis of storytelling provides insights into how scientific facts become relevant in cultural processes of meaning-making and are mobilized to reproduce or transform socioeconomic structures (Carr 2010; Wolfgram 2016). Such analysis can be linked to the core premise of STS scholarship—that science is always already culturally situated, contextualized, and mobilized (Moyer and Nguyen 2016). In this book I build upon medical anthropological scholarship on global health that is in conversation with this core premise of STS (Fassin 2012; more on this below; e.g., Adams 2016). And I link such perspectives to linguistic anthropological theorizations of storytelling and value.

Storytelling and Narrative

My analysis in this book draws from scholarship in linguistic anthropology on stories, narratives, and storytelling, focusing on storytelling as a key part of the process by which people imagine value systems unto being. The approach that I take is expansive and eclectic. There is a long anthropological tradition of the study of stories, narrative, and verbal art, alongside allied approaches in sociolinguistics, conversation analysis, and discourse analysis (see De Fina and Georgakopoulou 2015). One classic and still relevant theorization that informs everything written in this book is the idea that verbal art should be analyzed as not only a text (e.g., the words, phrases, and organization of a story) but also a performance (e.g., the social situation in which a story is told, the audience to which it is told, and the temporal unfolding of the story in the moment of its telling) (Bauman 1975; Ochs 2004). The history of the study of stories as text stretches back to at least the time of Aristotle, focusing things like the fundamental structure of a story and the connections between narratives and cognition (see De Fina and Georgakopoulou 2011, Chapter 1, for an overview). The study of narrative and storytelling as performance is more recent, including what has been termed "the narrative turn" in the 1980s (De Fina 2021).

Though some scholarship distinguishes storytelling (e.g., cultural traditions of telling myths, legends, folktales) from narratives (of personal experience), recent research argues that this distinction may not always be relevant (Falconi and Graber 2019: 2). Other work examines how plots may unfold across a range of social and communicative contexts including social media and other online spaces (e.g., De Fina and Perrino 2019). The blurring of the lines between story and narrative and the circulation of stories across contexts online and in person is evident in global health stories—for instance, when an epidemiologist at a symposium is recorded talking about what "we" (referring to an NPO) are doing to create and implement a health intervention in a low-income setting, and then this recording is posted on the NPO's YouTube channel.

Once I started thinking about the field of global health in terms of techno-optimistic stories, I found them seemingly everywhere—in YouTube videos, in glossy annual reports, and even as incipient stories in the ways that statistics are named and framed. In this book I probe the role that such stories, with their ability to emplot links between past, present, and future, played in the maintenance and transformation of scientific discourses of techno-optimism. I use these understandings of storytelling not only to understand the field of global health but also to provide insights about what it means to be human, especially how humans use storytelling to create and maintain systems of meaning—value systems—that guide actions amid the shaping constraints of larger socioeconomic, political, and historical forces.

The concept of imagination is central to my analysis. Philosopher Paul Ricoeur describes storytelling—and in particular, emplotment—as providing an entry point into the "kingdom of the *as if*" (Ricoeur 1984: 64). This sense of the subjunctive, of the way things could, should, or might be, is central to human value systems. Yet while narratives do have significance in processes of meaning-making meaning, they are also "articulations of the embodied struggle to morally be with oneself and others in the social world" (Zigon 2012: 204–205). Thus stories should not be assumed to be objective, comprehensive, or even necessarily accurate accounts of events that have occurred or even human experiences of those events (Ochs and Capps 2001: 45; Zigon 2012: 206). For the creation of value systems, the question of whether stories are accurate is less significant than the question of what stories do for people's imaginings.

In fact, the idea of imagination is an excellent pivot between theorizations of storytelling and theorizations of value. For instance, David Graeber (2001) writes,

> Value, I'll suggest, can best be seen… as the way in which actions become meaningful to the actor by being incorporated in some larger social totality—even if in many cases the totality in question exists primarily in the actor's *imagination.*
>
> (vii, emphasis added) (see Graeber 2013: 226)

Value systems result from processes through which human actions become associated with something larger—e.g., a community or a cause. But in everyday life this something larger often remains abstract, or, as Graeber puts it, imagined. And where better to look for the imagination than in storytelling, and in poetics, performance, and verbal art more generally?

The Anthropology of Value: A Semiotic Approach

In line with Graeber's definition, many contemporary anthropologists conceptualize value as

> the way different groups of people decide what is important, how that sense of importance manifests in objects and people, and, in turn, how those objects and people circulate, how they are cherished, used, and/or destroyed, as well as what happens when one regime of value meets the other.
>
> (Souleles, Archer, and Thaning 2023: 162)

Here, anthropology's holistic cross-cultural and historical perspective leads to a theory of value that is quite distinct from that of economics or philosophy. This perspective is rooted in classic anthropological research that documents and theorizes how pre-capitalist economic systems (primarily gift economies) operated according to ethical values: a person may give a neighbor, relative, or other acquaintance something they need with no expectation of immediate return, but over the long run a general system of reciprocity (organized around socioculturally specific ethical principles) shapes patterns of return on that gift (Mauss 2000 [1950]). More recent scholarship shows how such ethical value systems can persist, co-exist uneasily with, and be a source of capitalist value (Hutchinson 1992; Tsing 2013).

If value systems are not just about economics, an anthropological approach requires a theory broad enough to encompass multiple overlapping and sometimes conflicting ways of deciding what is important. Semiotics and linguistic anthropology provide tools to understand this phenomenon (e.g., Graber 2023; Cavanaugh and Shankar 2014). In this book, I employ Paul Kockelman's (2020) definition of value. He theorizes how distinct types of value (e.g., exchange value, use value, semiotic value) each adhere to the same general semiotic processes of creation, maintenance, and transformation. Kockelman defines value as "*a relation between agents mediated by a relation between entities*, where the agents need not be people and the entities need not be things" (6, emphasis in original). Or as he also puts it, relations between relations (3). For instance, he describes capitalist value as "a relation between people (say, factory owners and workers) mediated by a relation between things (say, means of production and labor power)" (5). Notably, in developing his theory, Kockelman examines a Mayan story. He discusses how that story produces and circulates multiple types of value; and he concludes that one value of stories is that they imaginatively constitute worlds—and also thus limit the scope of one's imagination in this constitution of worlds (101–104).

My analysis in this book suggests that the role of stories in defining value relations is bivalent. The construction of story plots (through emplotment) and the imbuing of these plots with ethical stances (through multimodal poetics) provides a vehicle for the reproduction and transformation of specific ideas and ideologies. At the same time, as stories become conventionalized (what linguistic anthropologists would call "entextualized") (Briggs and Bauman 1992), they may become objects of value in and of themselves—objects that can be commodified and/or exchanged as they are told and retold.

Here, storytelling is subject to the same sorts of opportunities and constraints as other forms of creative communication. Stories provide the chance to imagine something new into being. But to be meaningful to others and to circulate broadly, stories must—to some degree—reproduce the linguistic and cultural conventions of already existing stories (Lavie, Narayan, and Rosaldo 1993; Black 2008; Wilf 2012; Bakhtin 1986). In my analysis of global health storytelling in this book, the liberatory possibilities for creating health equity are limited by the conventions of stories—especially those stories told for powerful philanthropist audiences—leading to narratives in which a predictable cast of characters of elites from the global North enact technological solutions.

Stories and storytelling are crucial aspects of both scholarly and popular efforts at crafting optimistic futures, including futures that address the inequities of the past and present. Through emplotment, humans are able to articulate viewpoints on the time ahead, implicitly or explicitly connecting presents and pasts to possible futures. With this book, I hope to push global health to reimagine global health futures in ways that are more equitable in ways that global health practitioners hope to be. To do this requires an analysis and deconstruction of the stories that global health professionals currently tell, and the futures that these stories currently envision.

What's New about Global Health

Contemporary global health is dominated by NPOs that are overtly secular (Brown 2014; Addiss 2018).[9] Many of these NPOs rely on donations from philanthropists and corporations to fund their organizations; and NPO leaders tell particular sorts of stories that are designed to appeal to such donors. In this book, I address how this configuration—of persons, groups, institutions, and exchanges of resources (including the exchange of stories)—shapes global health priorities, actions, and the imaginative horizon of what is thought to be possible. While the dominance of NPOs is distinct in global health, this relatively new field has roots stretching back to the beginnings of the 20th century and beyond.

The term global health was first used in scientific literature in the 1940s, but the concept as it is now understood was not expanded upon until the 1990s (Packard 2016).[10] Still, the field is closely linked to its predecessors, including international health, colonial medicine, and missionary medicine (Greene et al. 2013; Packard 2016). In this context, anthropologists have been fairly critical about the field's novelty and distinctiveness. For instance, Vincanne Adams (2016) describes "the widely shared sentiment among many medical anthropologists who had devoted years to the work of 'international health' that 'global health' was itself a bit of a thief" (186). Similarly, Didier Fassin (2012) notes that many organizations and institutions have "created websites about activities that are not necessarily very distinct from what they had previously carried out under a different designation, such as public health, international health, health development, or health cooperation"; this leads Fassin to conclude that these activities "are not so much medical novelties as semiotic innovations. Technologies have evolved little, but the message is distinctive" (Fassin 2012: 101). This conclusion calls out for linguistic anthropological analysis, in particular an examination of how practitioners craft this distinct message online and in person.

Still, Fassin, Adams, and others describe key conceptual shifts that occurred from the 1990s to the 2010s. This included an increasing reliance on "data-driven" responses aided by complex logistical choreography—both of which were made possible by computer-aided technological innovations—which added to rather than replaced moralistic calls to action rooted in universalistic notions of humanity (Adams 2016). This was linked to a conceptualization of the global that is linguistically constructed through the localization—and thus exclusion—of professionals from low- and middle-income countries (Brada 2011, 2017).

The Shape of Contemporary Global Health

When I conducted a search for the phrase "global health" in historical and contemporary databases of American English, I found that rather than shifting over time, the term rapidly appears in these corpora just before the year 2000. In the Corpus of Historical American English (a collection of print sources such as magazines and newspapers from 1810–2009), my search returned seven results, six of which appear from 1999 onward. In the Corpus of Contemporary American English (a much larger database of online sources from 1990 to 2019), my search returned 833 hits, ninety-seven percent of which (811) appeared from 2000 onward.

This sudden rise in the use of the term "global health" matches an impressive increase in its financial support. In 1990, governmental sources and UN agencies provided and controlled the largest share of a total of 8.67 billion US dollars of funding for these activities (adjusted to 2014 dollars—see Figure 1.1). By 2018, this had increased to a total of forty-six billion dollars of funding (adjusted to 2024 dollars)—an almost five-fold increase in funding in nearly thirty years—with the largest share controlled by foundations and NPOs rather than governments or UN agencies (Figure 1.2). By 2020, with development banks contributing large amounts

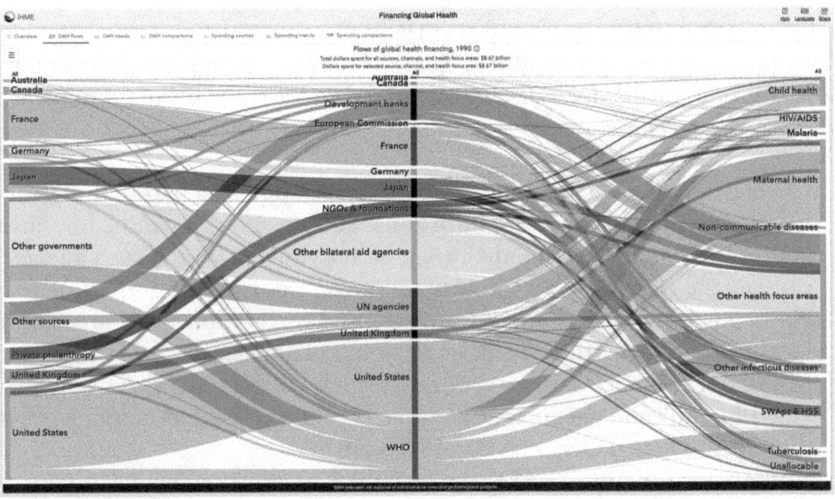

Figure 1.1 Flows of Global Health Financing, 1990.

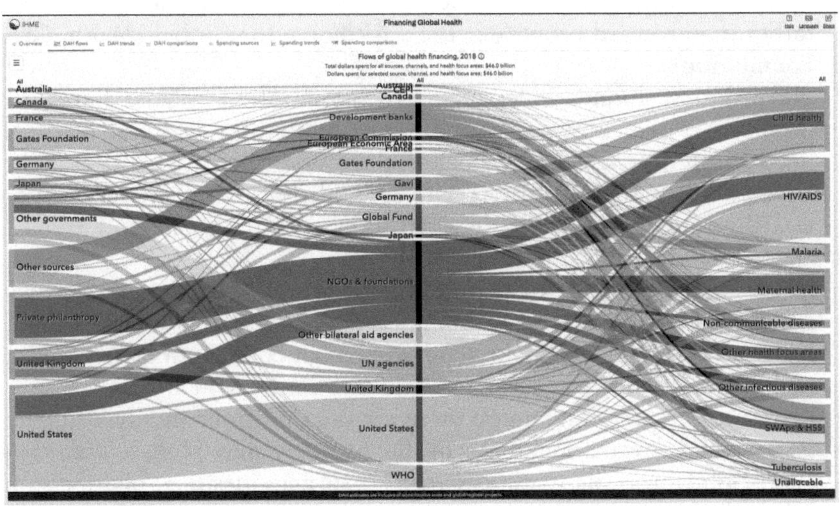

Figure 1.2 Flows of Global Health Financing, 2018. Screenshots from the Institute for Health Metrics and Evaluation data visualization website https://vizhub.healthdata.org/fgh/. Accessed 11/19/2024.

of money to responses to the COVID-19 pandemic, total funding for global health had increased to 67.5 billion dollars (adjusted to 2024 dollars—almost eight times as much as the 1990 funding level) (IHME 2024). Here, it is important to note that this massive funding increase occurred after governmental reductions in funding for health care in low-income countries—reductions that were part of the implementation of neoliberal development policies in the 1980s (discussed further in Chapter 2).

As this visualization of global health financing demonstrates, contemporary global health includes a dizzying range of types of institutions and organizations. These include:

- Governmental agencies: these are agencies funded by a national, state, or local government. Such organizations' actions are constrained by laws and policies that describe the range of activities in which such agencies can engage (e.g. CDC in the United States, the Georgia Department of Public Health [in the state of Georgia], and the National Department of Health in South Africa are all governmental agencies)
- Multilateral agencies: these are agencies whose funding is primarily provided by multiple national governments (e.g. the United Nations [UN], the World Health Organization [WHO])
- Secular and religious NPOs: often called non-governmental organizations in the United States, NPOs may have distinct legal standing in some countries (as they do in the United States) and reduced or eliminated taxes. Employees in NPOs may be paid very well, but the charter of these organizations is oriented toward some defined social good rather than toward profit (e.g. the Task Force for Global Health, CDC Foundation)
- Philanthropic foundations: these are organizations whose funding is primarily provided by one or more private donors. These are often defined as NGOs/NPOs, but I define them as being distinct from other NPOs because their priorities tend to be driven by one or several very wealthy contributors (e.g., the Soros Foundation, the Bill and Melinda Gates Foundation)
- Development banks: provide funding for projects that would otherwise not be able to be funded by commercial lenders. This includes multinational development banks funded through contributions of multiple national governments (e.g., the World Bank, the IMF)
- Corporations and companies: these are organizations that have a charter oriented toward making a profit, but they may include donations and/or philanthropic work as part of their activities (e.g. pharmaceutical companies)
- Universities: In recent years, numerous centers and programs have appeared with the aim of training public and global health professionals and also contributing directly to global health initiatives

Networks comprising several of these different types of organizations are often driven by funding and priorities of health professionals from high-income countries, while the targets of health interventions tend to be low- and middle-income countries or low-income communities within high-income countries. And as these economic distinctions largely follow from the relationship of former colonizers and colonized, global health also tends to involve White persons making decisions about the lives of people of the global majority (sometimes referred to as BIPOC [Black, Indigenous, and People of Color] in the United States)—though the field is changing in this regard and becoming more equitable. Such inequities are not unique to global health.

In this book, I focus especially on the Atlanta metropolitan area. Since the 1980s, former CDC employees and other public health specialists have created an impressive array of global health groups in Atlanta that include the Task Force for Global Health (the fourth largest NPO in the United States at the time I was writing the book) and CDC Foundation (a non-profit affiliated with CDC whose creation was authorized by congress in 1992). Other prominent global health players in the Atlanta area include the Carter Center (founded by former president Jimmy Carter and his wife, Rosalynn Carter), CARE, and Emory University.[11] A number of these Atlanta-based organizations enjoy close ties with the Bill and Melinda Gates Foundation, whose funding amounts so overwhelm those of other philanthropic organizations that the foundation profoundly shapes conversations in the field. In managing this wide range of institutions and interests, many of the global health professionals with whom I spoke favored what they called "public-private partnerships" that are designed to match governmental public health systems (which ideally provide authority, organization, and potential for long-term change) with the flexibility of action possible in private organizations and the funds provided by corporate donors. Examination of how Atlanta-area global health experts explain and discuss their work provides a much-needed window into global health in the global North.

Situating the Project: The Polymorphous Engagement of Studying Up

In 2016, I began the Global Health Discourses Project, focusing on the study of secular NPOs in the metropolitan Atlanta area. As mentioned, I found that global health NPO leaders were collegial, supportive of my general project, and willing to be interviewed, but were unwilling to open their organizations up to the scrutiny of participant observation. I would have to find alternative strategies to learn more about the field. In response, I shifted gears to focus my participant observation on aspects of everyday life in Decatur, Georgia, complemented by interviews, attendance at public events, and analysis of publicly available online materials.

Such an approach resonates with previous anthropological scholarship on how to study people in positions of power (Nader 1972). One noted challenge in these contexts is that researchers often lack access to the spaces in which power is made and remade (Ortner 2010). People from powerful socioeconomic backgrounds (and this includes many people who consider themselves to be middle class) often see few advantages to consenting to the kind of intensive opening-up of one's life to a researcher that is usually part of participant observation. This necessitates creative solutions. Hugh Gusterson (1997) suggests de-emphasizing participant observation and instead aiming for polymorphous engagement, by which he means "interacting with informants across a number of dispersed sites, not just in local communities, and sometimes in virtual form; and... collecting data eclectically from a disparate array of sources in many different ways" (116; see also Souleles 2018). In line with such work, my project draws from a range of methods to study global health discourses across distinct yet related sites.

As mentioned, living in Decatur, Georgia, it is difficult to avoid the world of global health. Many neighbors and friends work for CDC, whose headquarters are just a few miles away, or with the Task Force for Global Health, located in downtown Decatur, or at Emory University, about two miles from the city (and some have worked for all three). This is reflected in a statistic from the American Community Survey of the US Census Bureau: in Decatur, a staggering forty-three percent of city residents over age twenty-five have attained a graduate or professional degree (in comparison to thirteen percent in the state of Georgia as a whole).[12] I learned information that was important for this project in conversations at block parties, at neighborhood pubs, and while walking my children to and from school. My barber even helped with recruitment efforts by sharing my contact information with another client of his who was a CDC leader.

Beyond the Insider/Outsider Dichotomy

As a Decatur resident and fellow academic with an interest in global health, I am a semi-insider in this global health community. Anthropology has historically distinguished between the ethnographer who travels to conduct fieldwork in an unfamiliar place, on the one hand (making the "strange" into something "familiar"), and the ethnographer who conducts fieldwork in one's own home community, on the other (making the "familiar" into something "strange"); but this dichotomy is at best an oversimplification (Jacobs-Huey 2002; Abu-Lughod 1991; Narayan 1993). Even in the earliest anthropological research, ethnographers usually first appeared at field sites after those communities had encountered missionaries and colonial officials. In contemporary settings, researchers who come from far away and have little previous knowledge of a community are still often known entities to research participants in some respects. For instance, when I conducted research in South Africa I was new to the group of HIV patient-activists with whom I worked, but they knew numerous other American researchers and aid workers. At the same time, for those who study "their own" communities, to be an ethnographer means to gain and apply academic training that in some ways estranges oneself when working in one's home community. One may have some connections to a community that one studies (e.g., shared linguistic background, one parent or family member from a place) while still not being "from" there (see discussion in Mendoza-Denton 2008: 42–44). Ethnographers' backgrounds, identities, and connections to fieldwork communities are usually considerably more complex than the classic "familiar-strange" idea allows.

My previous experience suggests that the most productive approach to understanding the relationship between a researcher and a group of research participants is to contextualize our entanglements within an analysis of the larger socioeconomic forces and historical trends that shape the myriad of groups, organizations, and institutions relevant to a field site or field sites (Black and Riner 2022: 98; Narayan 1993). In my work, this has meant thinking expansively about my relationship to my neighbors and other Atlanta-based global health professionals in the context of universities, secular NPOs, government institutions, multilateral agencies, health activists, aid recipients, and community members across these varied sites (see also Marcus 1995 on multi-sited ethnography). This includes my positionality (as a white/Jewish, cisgender, heterosexual middle-class American man), which tends to align in various ways with the positionality of the majority of public and global health professionals that I have met in the Atlanta area (Goodman, Plepys, and Healton 2020).[13]

Methods and Ethics

Recognizing this partial alignment, in this book I draw primarily from my experiences in daily life in a community saturated by global health professionals, participant observation at public global health events in the Atlanta area, interviews with public and global health professionals, publicly available recordings taken from the YouTube pages of global health organizations, news stories about global health, and websites of global health organizations (including a content analysis and a social network analysis of how organizations' websites referred to other organizations). My analysis is also informed by my experience collaborating with global health scholar-practitioners from Costa Rica (who work with and train American global health students) and my previous fieldwork in South Africa (with research participants who were themselves entangled with practitioners from the global North).

When I was finishing fieldwork for this book, I pivoted to include information about responses to COVID-19. As the contours of the pandemic began to take shape in 2020, many neighbors were working from home, talking in the streets (outdoors to lessen exposure to the virus), and, crucially, talking extensively about public health. In such a context it was simple to bring up my research and to ask for neighbors' expert opinions about a range of subjects related to global health. In addition, I also had previously completed several distinct but related examinations of online global health content. In the Spring and Summer of 2017, I worked with Gabriela Alvarado[14] to analyze the process through which a Costa Rican global health organization created a new website. This included participant observation by Alvarado with that organization, as well as analysis of the new website content and an interview with the leader of the Costa Rican organization. The chapter based on this research that appears in this book is co-authored—something that reflects my collaboration with Costa Rican scholars and an equity-based approach to co-authorship and research. In Fall 2018, I also worked with five undergraduate student researchers—Kristina Ellis, Kathryn Leek, Scarlett Mayoralgo, Ana Marissa Rodriguez, and Savannah Setter—to carry out a qualitative thematic coding of the (very extensive) websites of six global health organizations (Africare, the Bill and Melinda Gates Foundation, CARE, the Task Force for Global Health, UNAIDS, and the World Health Organization). Student researcher Ellis also interviewed a person who had worked in global health for many years. In Spring 2019, I worked with Ally Chace, who was an MA student at the time, to complete a social network analysis of the website of the Task Force for Global Health. This entailed creating a list of all the partners/collaborators that the Task Force listed on their website, then going to the websites of all those partners/collaborators and listing all the organizations that those partners/collaborators listed on their websites (resulting in a list of 369 distinct organizations taken from 16 NPO websites). In 2020, I also completed an analysis of YouTube videos posted by three Atlanta-area organizations: the Task Force for Global Health, the CDC Foundation, and Child Health and Mortality Prevention Surveillance (CHAMPS) Health.

Finally, from 2016 to 2022, in addition to the interview I conducted with a Costa Rican global health professional and the interview Ellis conducted, I completed semi-structured interviews with six other global health professionals (eight interviews in total). Each of these interviews was with a person who specialized in a distinct facet of global health—for instance, a communications manager for an organization, the head of a special program or initiative, and a health communications specialist. The purpose of each of these interviews was not to provide generalizable data, but rather to learn about an expert's perspective on key aspects of global health discourse that I had identified through my other analysis.

Though ethical issues related to anonymity and confidentiality have been somewhat muted in this project as I am primarily dealing with public discourses, my growing awareness of how NPOs rely on their reputation and image in order to attract grant money and donations has meant that it is important that be cognizant of the potential for negative statements made in my work to harm an organization—not only the harm to the careers of global health professionals, but also the potential harm to target communities of health interventions. In other words, thinking about care for marginalized communities also entails attending to potential damage to the reputations of global health professionals and NPOs. I have worked to balance critique of problematic patterns in the narrative constitution of global health while also emphasizing that this is constructive critique aimed at improving global health and not aimed at any one particular organization.

A Note on "Doing Better" and "Decolonization"

Decolonization is one way to answer the question of how they (and we) might do better. Recently, this concept has gained traction among some in global health as it has in other fields and in popular discourses. In anthropology, the concept of decolonization can be traced back to work in Indigenous anthropology, Black feminist anthropology, and world anthropology—work in which "the 'coloniality'… Eurocentrism, and phallocentrism of much of hegemonic anthropology are problematized, and epistemic diversity, in its varied domestic and international permutations, is embraced as a matter of both principle and intellectual imperative" (Harrison 2016: 163). In the field of global health, calls to decolonize envision a future in which imbalances between professionals from low- and middle-income countries and those from high-income countries are "a thing of the past," with equity in academic authorship, decentralized and democratized knowledge platforms, an end to the notion that expertise flows from high-income countries to low- and middle-income countries, and "no dependence, only mutual training" (Abimbola and Pai 2020: 1628). Additionally, advocates note, to undo supremacy in global health will require responses to inequities in relationships *within* low-, middle-, and high-income countries (not just *between* low-/middle- and high-income countries), and further engagement with a critical understanding of the "sociostructural production of health" (Allotey and Reidpath 2021). Such an approach resonates with some of the critical perspectives of STS scholarship introduced above, insofar as both emphasize the significance of the culturally and socioeconomically situated nature of knowledge production. At key points throughout this book, I draw on work that is aligned with various approaches to decolonizing global health, anthropology, and academia in general.

What's Next?

In the remaining chapters, I examine three types of value (epistemic, ethical, and economic) that are central to contemporary global health and three linguistic/communicative phenomena (multimodal poetics, emplotment, and circulation) that are significant in the constitution of these values in storytelling. Though all make appearances throughout the book, each type of value and each phenomenon is emphasized in one of three chapters on values: ethical values are paired with multimodal poetics in Chapter 3; economic values are paired with circulation in Chapter 4; and epistemic values are paired with emplotment in Chapter 5. Before turning to this analysis, Chapter 2 discusses the history of global health in Atlanta, setting the stage for the rest of the book. And after the discussion of these values and communicative phenomena in Chapters 3–5, Chapter 6 provides a closer look at the process of creating global health stories during a website redesign process. Finally, Chapter 7 concludes this book, drawing on recent anthropological scholarship to suggest ways to better align global health storytelling with the values of equity and decolonization that global health professionals and organizations espouse.

In Chapter 2, I introduce Atlanta as a global health city, focusing in particular on the metropolitan area as one of the birthplaces of techno-optimistic, secular, NPO-driven global health. I introduce key organizations and individuals that shape the field in Atlanta, and who will be featured throughout the remainder of the book. In addition to published histories, I analyze a treasure trove of materials from the Global Health Chronicles, a website that provides a lightly curated selection of archival photographs, letters, and recorded interviews with public health leaders from the beginnings of CDC onward. The picture that emerges through my analysis is a city where private philanthropy has long been intertwined with public health, and where the field was thus poised to adapt to neoliberal economic policies of the 1980s—policies that stripped international health efforts of governmental funding while simultaneously reducing the ability of low-income nations to offer socialized health care. The solutions to this socioeconomic situation devised in Atlanta would reverberate throughout the world of global health over the next forty years.

In Chapter 3, I shift to a discussion of contemporary Atlanta, focusing on how the ethical values of global health are constituted through storytelling online and in person. I re-examine what is often assumed to be a dichotomy between approaches to health rooted in notions of cost-effectiveness, on the one hand, and approaches rooted in notions of health as a human right, on the other. Drawing from an analysis of interview data and recorded public events with global health professionals, I suggest that ethical values demonstrated by those associated with secular

NPOs are more complex and pragmatically oriented toward the effort to provide care to those who need it but are otherwise unable to pay for it. I discuss how global health stories deploy the concepts of collaboration and partnership in the constitution of this pragmatic ethics as they tell techno-optimistic stories, but also how the multimodal poetics of these stories link collaboration and partnership to racialized indexes of care, in some ways undermining the very ethical principles that global health professionals seek to enact.

In Chapter 4 I answer the question of why global health stories might deploy these racialized indexes of care despite their shortcomings, focusing on how stories circulate and become associated with philanthropists. In my discussion I primarily analyze public-facing communication of Atlanta-based NPOs. While Chapters 3 and 5 examine how values are constituted in stories and their telling, Chapter 4 focuses on the values associated with the circulation of these techno-optimistic stories and the monetary impact of this circulation. For ethical values to be transferrable to donors, they must be embedded in stories—ideally in well-told stories performed by virtuosic storytellers. Here, I identify the values of transparency, successfulness, and virtuosity as key concepts for understanding the economics of global health storytelling. My analysis demonstrates that the most transportable stories may reinforce harmful stereotypes about who (in terms of race, gender, nationality, class) tend to be the targets and implementers of global health interventions. In this way, the aesthetics of virtuosic global health storytelling tend to reinforce existing inequities between global health professionals based in high-income countries and communities that are the targets of health interventions.

In Chapter 5, I examine how epistemic values are constituted in global health through an exploration of the narrative emplotment of techno-optimism during the COVID-19 pandemic in the Atlanta metropolitan area and the United States as a whole. After identifying five building blocks of techno-optimistic plots in global health stories, I analyze how the phrase "flatten the curve" entered into circulation in public health discussions about the pandemic in 2020, suggesting how this concept became imbued with techno-optimistic value. Next, I turn to a discussion of dueling editorials about reopening the schools in Decatur, Georgia, written by public health professionals who lived in the city. This discussion introduces the idea of global health antiheroes: story protagonists that focus on socioeconomic inequities and structural changes and thus that do not fit the mold of the heroes that so often pervade global health stories. I then turn to arguments about the efficacy of alternative medical treatments, including ivermectin and hydroxychloroquine.

This analysis shows how the building blocks of techno-optimism were utilized by promoters of these medically ineffective treatments, suggesting that a narrow dismissal of these stories as "anti-science" may have hampered the ability to counter this disinformation. Finally, I describe public and global health professionals' emphasis on vaccines as the only viable solution to the pandemic, setting the stage for a nuanced discussion about science, technology, and low-tech common-sense public health actions that never took place due to their conflict with neoliberal capitalism. This showcases how techno-optimism becomes a narrative through-line that underlies many diverse discursive developments, including some sometimes described as "anti-science."

In Chapter 6 I write with co-author Gabriela Alvarado to provide a case study focused on the creation of a global health website. This chapter is based on participant observation with a Costa Rican educational global health organization as that organization's leaders redesigned their website. Though the organization was based in Costa Rica, the analysis offered here is nonetheless relevant to the study of global health in Atlanta because academic global health professionals in the United States (including Atlanta) were the NPO's main imagined audience as they worked through the redesign process. Indeed, NPO leaders had traveled to Atlanta to promote their organization and later worked with professors in Atlanta and in other US cities. The analysis we offer in this chapter describes how epistemic, ethical, and economic values are mediatized—that is, mediated and simultaneously commodified—in the process of creating a digital infrastructure for the circulation of global health stories. We also provide some insights into difficulties faced by global health professionals from low- and middle-income countries. They often balance the need to tell techno-optimistic stories to attract resources from high-income countries, on the one hand, with the moral obligation to emphasize the significance of global health's structural intervention antiheroes and advocate for truly transformative care in low-income settings, on the other hand.

Chapter 7, the conclusion, provides a summary of key points of the book within the framework of attempting to answer the question of how the future of global health might be reimagined by changing specific components of how stories are told in the field. In suggesting partial answers to this question, the chapter draws from contemporary medical anthropology research on topics such as biomedicalization, the social determinants of health, and the concept of accompaniment. The book then ends by summarizing the theoretical contributions offered in the text, synthesizing scholarship from economic, linguistic, and medical anthropology to present a new model of the role of storytelling in the constitution of human value systems.

Notes

1 https://www.usatoday.com/story/news/health/2020/03/10/coronavirus-georgia-residents-cdc-headquarters-safe-messonnier/4929882002/. Accessed 1/12/23.
2 I am uncertain where this phrase originated. I found it on the Emory University Rollins School of Public Health webpage.
3 https://www.cdc.gov/about/priorities/why-is-addressing-sdoh-important.html. Accessed 3/1/24.
4 Despite a number of scholarly statements on the matter, it is unclear precisely what the difference is between the terms NGO and NPO. In this book, I use NPO for two reasons: first, to highlight the need for these organizations to constantly fundraise and/or get grants; and, second, to emphasize anthropological theorizations of governmentality that argue that the transition away from the use of formal government institutions (e.g., public health departments) to administer healthcare and other services does not mean *less* governance, but rather means a shift in governance away from elected officials to corporate and NPO leaders (Biehl 2006; Ferguson and Gupta 2002).
5 I sometimes use the terms global North and global South—a theorization that has entered into popular discourses—because these terms are a convenient shorthand for not only the wealth disparities between former colonizer countries/former colonized countries but also the power dynamics that accompany these disparities. More often, however, I simply use the categories defined by the United Nations of low-income, middle-income, and high-income countries (or low-, middle-, and high-income settings), because I feel that the intellectual frameworks associated with global North/ global South oversimplify the complex dynamics of wealth and power dynamics within low-, middle-, and high-income countries.
6 This project was approved by the Georgia State University IRB and research was conducted in accordance with IRB rules, guidelines, and approvals.
7 It is common practice to refer to not only medical doctors but also PhDs as doctors. In this book, for ease of reference this book uses "doctor" and the pronominal abbreviation "Dr." to identify medical doctors in particular.
8 There is an entire subfield of health communication research, but in that work the study of stories is primarily oriented toward how to best communicate medical knowledge and health recommendations to the public, rather than a critical analysis of how knowledge is produced, how it circulates, and to what ends.
9 I say overtly because many global health organizations, especially those based in the United States, have ethical antecedents rooted in missionary medicine (Brown 2014). Furthermore, many contemporary practitioners are motivated, at least in part, by spiritual factors to do the work that they do (Addiss 2015). I discuss this further in Chapter 3.
10 For a comprehensive discussion of the history of global health, see Packard 2016.
11 Here I would like to note that I seem to focus especially on the Task Force for Global Health in this book; this is not because I have singled that NPO out. Rather, it is simply because the Task Force has made more of their work and discussions about their work available to the public.
12 https://data.census.gov/table?tid=ACSDP5Y2021.DP02&g=0400000US13_1600000US1322052. Accessed 1/12/23.
13 https://cghi.org/women-in-global-health-georgia-chapter/.

14 Alvarado, a Costa Rican student who was working toward her MA in anthropology at Georgia State University at the time, had previously earned an MD in Costa Rica and a master's in public health, and had interned at a global health organization in Atlanta. She now holds a PhD in Policy Studies earned at the Pardee RAND Graduate School.

References

Abimbola, Seye, and Madhukar Pai. 2020. "Will Global Health Survive its Decolonization?" *The Lancet* 396 (10263): 1627–1628.

Abu-Lughod, Lila. 1991. "Writing Against Culture." In *Recapturing Anthropology*, edited by Richard Fox, 137–162. Santa Fe, NM: School of American Research.

Adams, Vincanne. 2016. "What Is Critical Global Health?" *Medicine Anthropology Theory* 3 (2): 186–197.

Addiss, David. 2018. "Spiritual Themes and Challenges in Global Health." *Journal of Medical Humanities* 39 (3): 337–348.

Allotey, Pascale, and Daniel D. Reidpath. 2021. "Undoing Supremacy in Global Health Will Require More than Decolonisation." *The Lancet* 397 (10279): 1058.

Arnold, Lynnette, Jennifer R. Guzmán, Emily Avera, and Anna I. Corwin, eds. Forthcoming. *Language and Health in Action*. New York: Oxford University Press.

Avle, Seyram, Cindy Lin, Jean Hardy, and Silvia Lindtner. 2020. "Scaling Techno-Optimistic Visions." *Engaging Science, Technology, and Society* 6: 237–254.

Bakhtin, Mikhail. 1986. "The Problem of Speech Genre." In *Speech Genres and Other Essays*, edited by Caryl Emerson and Michael Holquist, 60–102. Austin: University of Texas Press.

Bauman, Richard. 1975. "Verbal Art as Performance." *American Anthropologist* 77 (2): 290–311.

Benton, Adia. 2015. *HIV Exceptionalism: Development Through Disease in Sierra Leone*. Minneapolis, MN: University of Minnesota Press.

Berg, Ulla D., and Ana Y. Ramos-Zayas. 2015. "Racializing Affect: A Theoretical Proposition." *Current Anthropology* 56 (5): 654–677.

Berlant, Laura. 2011. *Cruel Optimism*. Durham, NC: Duke University Press.

Biehl, João. 2006. "Pharmaceutical Governance." In *Global Pharmaceuticals: Ethics, Markets, Practices*, edited by Adriana Petryna, Andrew Lakoff, and Arthur Kleinman, 206–239. Durham, NC: Duke University Press.

Black, Steven P. 2008. "Creativity and Learning Jazz: The Practice of "Listening"." *Mind, Culture, and Activity* 15 (4): 279–295.

Black, Steven P., and Robin Conley Riner. 2022. "Care as a Methodological Stance: Research Ethics in Linguistic Anthropology." In *Research Methods in Linguistic Anthropology*, edited by Sabina M. Perrino and Sonya E. Pritzker, 97–123. New York: Bloomsbury.

Brada, Betsey Behr. 2011. "'Not *Here*': Making the Spaces and Subjects of 'Global Health' in Botswana." *Culture, Medicine, and Psychiatry* 35 (2): 285–312.

Brada, Betsey Behr. 2017. "Exemplary or Exceptional? The Production and Dismantling of Global Health in Botswana." In *Global Health and Geographical Imaginaries*, edited by Clare Herrick and David Reubi, 40–53. New York: Routledge.

Briggs, Charles L. 2020. "Beyond the Linguistic/Medical Anthropology Divide: Retooling Anthropology to Face COVID-19." *Medical Anthropology* 39 (7): 563–572.

Briggs, Charles L. 2021. *Unlearning: Rethinking Poetics, Pandemics, and the Politics of Knowledge*. Louisville, CO: University Press of Colorado.

Briggs, Charles L., and Richard Bauman. 1992. "Genre, Intertextuality, and Social Power." *Journal of Linguistic Anthropology* 2 (2): 131–172.

Briggs, Charles L., and Paja Faudree. 2016. "Communicating Bodies: New Juxtapositions of Linguistic and Medical Anthropology." *Anthropology News* 2016 (57): e7–e8.

Briggs, Charles L., and Clara Mantini-Briggs. 2003. *Stories in the Time of Cholera: Racial Profiling During a Medical Nightmare*. Berkeley: University of California Press.

Briggs, Charles L., and Clara Mantini-Briggs. 2016. *Tell Me Why My Children Died: Rabies, Indigenous Knowledge, and Communicative Justice*. Durham, NC: Duke University.

Brown, Peter J. 2014. "Religion and Global Health." In *Religion as a Social Determinant of Global Health*, edited by Ellen Idler, 273–297. Oxford: Oxford University Press.

Büyüm, Ali Murad, Cordelia Kenney, Andrea Koris, Laura Mkumba, and Yadurshini Raveendran. 2020. "Decolonising Global Health: If Not Now, When?" *BMJ Global Health* 5 (8): 1–4.

Carr, E. Summerson. 2010. "Enactments of Expertise." *Annual Review of Anthropology* 39: 17–32.

Cavanaugh, Jillian R., and Shalini Shankar. 2014. "Producing Authenticity in Global Capitalism: Language, Materiality, and Value." *American Anthropologist* 116 (1): 51–64.

Closser, Svea. 2012. "'We Can't Give Up Now': Global Health Optimism and Polio Eradication in Pakistan." *Medical Anthropology* 31 (5): 385–403.

Crane, Johanna Tayloe. 2013. *Scrambling for Africa: AIDS, Expertise, and the Rise of American Global Health Science*. Ithaca, NY: Cornell University Press.

De Fina, Anna. 2021. "Doing Narrative Analysis from a Narratives as Practices Perspective." *Narrative Inquiry* 31 (1): 49–71.

De Fina, Anna, and Alexandra Georgakopoulou. 2011. *Analyzing Narrative: Discourse and Sociolinguistic Perspectives*. New York: Cambridge University Press.

De Fina, Anna, and Alexandra Georgakopoulou, eds. 2015. *The Handbook of Narrative Analysis*. Malden, MA: Wiley Blackwell.

De Fina, Anna, and Sabina Perrino, eds. 2019. *Storytelling in the Digital World*. Philadelphia, PA: John Benjamins.

Ellis, Nicquel Terry, and Jayne O"Donnell. 2020. "War on Coronavirus: Residents in Suburban Atlanta Town Find Comfort Near CDC Headquarters." *USA Today*. Accessed 3/4/2022. https://www.usatoday.com/story/news/health/2020/03/10/coronavirus-georgia-residents-cdc-headquarters-safe-messonnier/4929882002/.

Falconi, Elizabeth, and Kathryn Graber. 2019. "Ethnographic Approaches to Storytelling as Narrative Practice." In *Storytelling as Narrative Practice: Ethnographic Approaches to the Tales We Tell*, edited by Elizabeth Falconi and Kathryn Graber, 1–24. Boston, MA: Brill.

Fassin, Didier. 2012. "That Obscure Object of Global Health." In *Medical Anthropology at the Intersections*, edited by Marcia C. Inhorn and Emily A. Wentzell, 95–115. Durham, NC: Duke University Press.

Ferguson, James, and Akhil Gupta. 2002. "Spatializing States: Toward an Ethnography of Neoliberal Governmentality." *American Ethnologist* 29 (4): 981–1002.

Goodman, Melody S., Christine M. Plepys, and Cheryl G. Healton. 2020. "Racial/Ethnic Diversity in Academic Public Health: 20-Year Update." *Public Health Reports* 135 (1): 74–81. https://doi.org/10.1177/0033354919887747.

Graber, Kathryn E. 2023. "Textures of Value: Tactility, Experience, and Exclusion in the Cashmere Commodity Chain." *Economic Anthropology* 10 (2): 186–196.

Graeber, David. 2001. *Toward an Anthropological Theory of Value: the False Coin of Our Own Dreams*. New York: Palgrave.

Graeber, David. 2013. "It Is Value That Brings Universes Into Being." *HAU: Journal of Ethnographic Theory* 3 (2): 219–243.

Greene, Jeremy, Marguerite Thorp Basilico, Heidi Kim, and Paul Farmer. 2013. "Colonial Medicine and Its Legacies." In *Reimagining Global Health: An Introduction*, edited by Paul Farmer, Jim Yong Kim, Arthur Kleinman, and Matthew Basilico, 33–73. Los Angeles: University of California Press.

Gusterson, Hugh. 1997. "Studying Up Revisited." *POLAR: Political and Legal Anthropology Review* 20 (1): 114–119.

Hall-Clifford, Rachel. 2024. *Underbelly: Childhood Diarrhea and the Hidden Local Realities of Global Health*. Durham, NC: Duke University Press.

Harrison, Fay V. 2016. "Theorizing in Ex-Centric Sites." *Anthropological Theory* 16 (2–3): 160–176.

Harvey, David. 2005. *A Brief History of Neoliberalism*. New York: Oxford University Press.

Hutchinson, Sharon E. 1992. "The Cattle of Money and the Cattle of Girls among the Nuer, 1930–83." *American Ethnologist* 19 (2): 294–316.

IHME, (Institute for Health Metrics and Evaluation). 2024. *Financing Global Health Visualization*. Seattle: IHME, University of Washington. https://vizhub.healthdata.org/fgh/. Accessed 11/19/2024.

Jacobs-Huey, Lanita. 2002. "The Natives Are Gazing and Talking Back: Reviewing the Problematics of Positionality, Voice, and Accountability Among "Native" Anthropologists." *American Anthropologist* 104 (3): 791–804.

Keshavjee, Salmaan. 2014. *Blind Spot: How Neoliberalism Infiltrated Global Health*. Berkeley: University of California Press.

Kockelman, Paul. 2020. *Kinds of Value: An Experiment in Modal Anthropology*. Chicago, IL: Prickly Paradigm Press.

Kofman, Ava. 2018. Bruno Latour, the Post-Truth Philosopher, Mounts a Defense of Science. *The New York Times Magazine*. Accessed 2/25/2022.

Latour, Bruno, and Steve Woolgar. 1987 [1979]. *Laboratory Life: The Construction of Scientific Facts*. Princeton, NJ: Princeton University Press.

Lavie, Smadar, Kirin Narayan, and Renato Rosaldo, eds. 1993. *Creativity/ Anthropology*. Ithaca, NY: Cornell University Press.

Marcus, George. 1995. "Ethnography in/of the World System: The Emergence of Multi-Sited Ethnography." *Annual Review of Anthropology* 24: 95–117.
Mauss, Marcel. 2000 [1950]. *The Gift: The Form and Reason for Exchange in Archaic Societies*. Translated by W. D. Halls. New York: Norton.
Mei, Yuyang. 2017. "Neoliberal Optimism: Applying Market Techniques to Global Health." *Medical Anthropology* 36 (4): 381–395.
Mendoza-Denton, Norma. 2008. *Homegirls: Language and Cultural Practice among Latina Youth Gangs*. Malden, MA: Wiley-Blackwell.
Moyer, Eileen, and Vinh-Kim Nguyen. 2016. "Is the 21st Century the Age of Biomedicalization?" *Medicine Anthropology Theory* 3 (1): i–vii.
Nader, Laura. 1972. "Up the Anthropologist: Perspectives Gained From Studying Up." In *Reinventing Anthropology*, edited by Dell Hymes, 284–311. New York: Pantheon Books.
Narayan, Kirin. 1993. "How Native Is a "Native" Anthropologist?" *American Anthropologist* 95: 671–685.
Ochs, Elinor. 2004. "Narrative Lessons." In *A Companion to Linguistic Anthropology*, edited by Alessandro Duranti, 269–289. Malden, MA: Blackwell Publishers.
Ochs, Elinor, and Lisa Capps. 2001. *Living Narrative: Creating Lives in Everyday Storytelling*. Cambridge, MA: Harvard University Press.
Ochs, Elinor, Patrick Gonzales, and Sally Jacoby. 1996. "When I Come Down I'm in a Domain State: Talk, Gesture, and Graphic Representation in the Interpretive Activity of Physicists." In *Interaction and Grammar*, edited by Elinor Ochs, Emanuel Schegloff and Sandra A. Thompson, 328–369. Cambridge: Cambridge University Press.
Ortner, Sherry B. 2010. "Access: Reflections on Studying Up in Hollywood." *Ethnography* 11 (2): 211–233.
Ortner, Sherry B. 2016. "Dark Anthropology and Its Others." *HAU: Journal of Ethnographic Theory* 6 (1): 47–73.
Packard, Randall M. 2016. *A History of Global Health: Interventions into the Lives of Other Peoples*. Baltimore, MD: Johns Hopkins University Press.
Ricoeur, Paul. 1984. *Time and Narrative*. Chicago, IL: University of Chicago Press.
Souleles, Daniel. 2018. "How to Study People who do not Want to be Studied: Practical Reflections on Studying Up." *POLAR: Political and Legal Anthropology Review* 41 (S1): 51–68.
Souleles, Daniel Scott, Matthew Archer, and Morten Sørensen Thaning. 2023. "Introduction to Special Issue: Value, Values, and Anthropology." *Economic Anthropology* 10 (2): 162–168.
Tsing, Anna. 2013. "Sorting Out Commodities: How Capitalist Value Is Made Through Gifts." *HAU: Journal of Ethnographic Theory* 3 (1): 21–43.
Wilf, Eitan. 2012. "Rituals of Creativity: Tradition, Modernity, and the 'Acoustic Unconscious' in a U.S. Collegiate Jazz Music Program." *American Anthropologist* 114 (1): 32–44.
Wolfgram, Matthew. 2016. "Science Talk and Scientific Reference." *Annual Review of Anthropology* 45: 33–44.
Zigon, Jarrett. 2012. "Narratives." In *A Companion to Moral Anthropology*, edited by Didier Fassin, 204–220. Malden, MA: Wiley-Blackwell.

2 Making Health Global in Atlanta

A History

In a promotional video posted on YouTube in 2017, two of the most significant figures in contemporary global health sit at a table in a library, books surrounding the two on shelves and artfully placed on the table itself.[1] Both of these figures are older white men with gray hair and glasses dressed in business attire. One is Bill Gates, the billionaire founder of Microsoft and the Bill and Melinda Gates Foundation—one of the largest charitable organizations in the world. Gates, who is wearing dark gray dress slacks and a beige collared shirt with the top button opened, leans back in his chair. The other person sitting at the table is Dr. William (Bill) Foege—former Centers for Disease Control and Prevention (CDC) director and founder of the Task Force for Global Health in Decatur. Perched at attention on the left, Foege is wearing a dark suite with a light blue-collared shirt and yellow tie. This video is posted to Gates' YouTube account and is titled "Heroes in the Field: Dr. Bill Foege."

In the video, Gates describes how he began to work with Foege in the mid to late 1990s, and how Foege then became a senior medical adviser for the Bill and Melinda Gates Foundation in 1999. Gates explains to Foege, "we had money to spend, but we were so naïve about what global health was, and you came with your wisdom, your experience, and it was the start of kind of a perfect relationship." This relationship would be emulated by others such as Mark Zuckerberg and George Soros, both of whom have used large private donations from the world's wealthiest individuals to fund global health non-profit organizations (NPOs). The relationship between Gates and Foege also solidified Atlanta's key position in the emerging field of global health in the early 2000s.

In the video, Gates states a public health factoid—that the mosquito is actually the most dangerous animal in the world because it is a vector for so many diseases (he mentions efforts to eradicate malaria, which is transmitted by mosquito). And he says that smallpox eradication, which Foege spearheaded, is "to this day the greatest health achievement ever," noting that people have been coming to Foege to ask for advice ever since. Gates

DOI: 10.4324/9781003561019-2

concludes by saying, "We've got science on our side, [and] we've got morality on our side"—in other words, epistemic and ethical values. He leaves out the third type of value (economic values) discussed in this book, but with Gates' status as one of the wealthiest philanthropists in the world, the monetary aspect of the arrangement is fairly clear. How did global health arrive at this configuration, particularly in Atlanta?

While previous scholarship has discussed global health's historical antecedents in great detail (Packard 2016; McGoey 2015; e.g., Greene et al. 2013), there is little scholarship that addresses the part played by Atlanta in that history. Yet the city's role in the development of contemporary global health has been significant. It was in Atlanta in the mid-1980s that Dr. Foege helped spearhead what is now known as the selective primary healthcare movement. This movement responded to significant reductions in governmental funding that Foege himself was forced to oversee as CDC director during the first years of Ronald Reagan's presidency. The selective primary healthcare movement shifted international efforts from the provision of holistic care for all to the provision of a limited suite of health services with a focus on children. One NPO that emerged during this shift, the Task Force for Child Survival (later renamed the Task Force for Global Health), was later at the forefront of the global health transition from governmental to philanthropic funding, public-private partnerships, and data-driven interventions, features that characterize contemporary global health. This was especially the case after Dr. Foege began to work with Bill Gates in the late 1990s. As this chapter will explore, Atlanta is not just a "global health capital"; the region has also played a central role in the historical development of the contemporary field of global health.

In addition to a published works on the history of public and global health in Atlanta, this chapter draws from a unique resource: the Global Health Chronicles (GHC, http://globalhealthchronicles.com). The GHC is a collection of historical materials and oral histories made publicly available online by the David J. Sencer CDC Museum and the Emory Center for Digital Scholarship (a veritable treasure for scholars). While the site describes itself as "public health archives," it is a curated display rather than a complete collection of all records. For this reason, this chapter treats the collection as itself shaped by the overarching story that CDC tells about its history. Like the other online materials (e.g., websites, videos) examined in this book, then, the analysis of the GHC yields a discussion of the values that the organization that produced it are putting on display. This chapter outlines the story that global health leaders tell about the development of key epistemic, ethical, and economic values in global health, discussing pivotal moments that contributed to the making of Atlanta as a global health hub. The chapter also introduces many of the organizations now involved in global health in the city, while describing how previous agendas and frameworks continue to impact contemporary work.

1930s–1940s: Mr. Anonymous and Philanthropy in Atlanta

It was in the 1930s that the forces that would shape CDC and its global health NPO offspring in Atlanta began to emerge. When sifting through the GHC's ample collection of materials from this time period, one name stands out from the rest: Robert Winship Woodruff. A search of the entire GHC collection for "Woodruff" yields a staggering 108 results. Woodruff's support as a powerful public figure in Atlanta, Georgia, and the United States helped the nascent governmental organization along at several key moments. This began with his early interest and funding of anti-malaria efforts in south Georgia.

To those familiar with the history of Atlanta or the names of museums and parks around the city, Woodruff's prominence may not seem surprising. After his father and other wealthy businessmen purchased Coca-Cola, Woodruff became president of the company and stayed in that role from 1923 until 1954. His philanthropic efforts began during that time period, and he remained a leading philanthropist in Atlanta long afterward. In downtown Atlanta, there is a Woodruff Park near Georgia State University and a Woodruff Arts Center (both named in his honor after his death), as well as a Robert W. Woodruff Library at the Atlanta University Center Consortium.[2] At Emory University there are several Woodruff-named centers and buildings (a library, a residential center, a health sciences center, and a physical education center)—many of which seem to be connected to a 105 million dollar donation to the university in 1979 (with later gifts from the Woodruff Foundation coming to a total of more than 500 million dollars).[3]

By the time of his death in 1985, Woodruff, his family, and Coca-Cola had established five foundations worth more than 500 million dollars (Barnes 1985).[4] The disjuncture of the head of a company whose products contribute significantly to childhood obesity, diabetes, and other health ailments promoting health interventions is notable, though the extent of these links did not become widely known until after Woodruff's death the 1990s. The Atlanta History Center describes Woodruff as having "held great influence" in Atlanta; "yet, he used his influence behind-the-scenes and donated money anonymously." Woodruff even gained the nickname "Mr. Anonymous." As a speech act, use of this name is paradoxical in the sense that people had to know that Woodruff was donating money in order to call him Mr. Anonymous, so that in a certain sense he could not have been anonymous. It is likely that he tried to remain anonymous in at least some cases, but other people revealed his generosity. This fits a general pattern in philanthropy, in which wealthy donors may disavow credit for or avoid celebration of their efforts, motivated by an ethical feeling that they are simply doing the right thing by donating; but recipient organizations may gain benefit from association with the name of the donor (this is discussed more in Chapter 4) (Harvey, Gordon, and Maclean 2021).

Woodruff had become a champion of health causes by 1937. After his mother died as a result of cancer, Woodruff established a cancer center at Emory University Hospital to honor her.[5] Here and throughout his philanthropy, I wonder how much of Robert Woodruff's efforts were influenced or directed by his spouse. Unfortunately, the gender norms of the time seem to have resulted in the erasure of much of Nell Woodruff's impact on the family's health philanthropy decision-making process. However, it is notable that Nell Woodruff studied nursing and served in the American Red Cross during World War I and World War II. When she is mentioned in available historical documents, websites, and publications, she is described as a "longtime leader in nursing and health fields" who served as a US delegate to the World Health Assemblies in 1954 and 1955.[6] The School of Nursing at Emory is named after her.

The Most Dangerous Animal on Earth

In addition to the Emory Cancer center, Robert Woodruff's interest in health causes included efforts combating malaria that date back to the early 1930s. Though the *anopheles* mosquito was identified as the animal vector for malaria transmission at beginning of the 20th century, the disease was still endemic in the South in the 1930s. After purchasing a large plantation in southwest Georgia to be a hunting preserve, named Ichuaway, Woodruff learned that malaria was widespread in the area. In published work about this historical moment, much is made of Woodruff's response: he generously purchased enough quinine to treat every resident of the county where the plantation was located and hired two nurses to distribute the medication (Etheridge 1992: 3). However, less is said about the fact that the plantation was "also a working farm complete with tenants working for shares."[7] I sometimes think about how these sharecroppers might have responded to Woodruff's top-down malaria-control efforts. Were residents given a choice about whether or not to be treated? If they were, did they feel obligated to participate in light of their socioeconomic position? Were there any efforts to respond to local cultural models that may have led residents to understand malaria differently? It would certainly be in keeping with public health efforts of the time period—both in the United States and abroad—for residents to be coerced into treatment (Packard 2016: ch. 1). Though nothing about the approach taken is mentioned in any available sources, this absence is itself an indication of the ways that cultural difference, economic distinctions, and power differentials were often treated as external to scientific medical interventions.

In the GHC, there is a collection of twenty-six letters and memorandums from 1938 to 1952, which include forty-eight pages of correspondence to, from, and about Robert Woodruff with regard to his anti-malaria efforts. Many letters to Woodruff are from Coca-Cola's medical advisor, Dr. Glenville Giddens, who was simultaneously the director of mosquito-control projects for the Georgia Power Company. Giddens was a close collaborator of Woodruff's on several public health efforts. Letters from Giddens include estimates of expenses, a few overt requests for funds, and reports on initiatives that seem to have been funded or suggested by Woodruff. There were also carefully worded implicit recommendations for Woodruff's funding, attention, or support, such as "The attached memorandum was prepared by the Georgia Department of Public Health... It struck me as being rather carefully thought out and practical in its application. I thought you might be interested in seeing a copy."[8]

Reading through this correspondence, I see the outlines of a social network of well-placed, powerful, wealthy White men linked to Coca-Cola and Emory University (what has sometimes derogatorily been called a "good old boys club"). While global health has diversified a great deal since the mid-20th century, certain aspects of this network have persisted. For instance, many global health professionals who are successful in their careers are connected to Emory. However, recent efforts have been made to make the field more inclusive in the Atlanta metropolitan region, including the creation of a group called the Georgia Global Health Alliance (GGHA)—an NPO that was the brainchild of Bill Foege. The GGHA was established in 2002 but not truly developed until 2013 and beyond.[9]

In an interview conducted in 1966, entomologist and epidemiologist Dr. Melvin Goodwin (who is an author of some correspondence with Woodruff) talks about Robert Woodruff's philosophy relating to efforts to control malaria at the south Georgia hunting preserve:

Excerpt 1: The Real Impact

> Goodwin: Many foundations are developed and much research is done in the medical field because someone visualizes the problem and the need for control. But to Mr. Woodruff, I think, this was always a very personal matter. He saw the people on the plantation who were suffering from malaria. He saw the real impact of hookworm disease. His philosophy—and one that I certainly share—seemed to be that research is more meaningful when the application of the efforts can

> be anticipated. Development of control programs is not complete until they are evaluated under operational conditions.[10]

Here, Goodwin articulates a forward-thinking, imaginative orientation to medical research (e.g., "when the application of the efforts can be anticipated"). His is essentially a statement about values, namely, that medical research is more valuable when it can be tied to a health intervention. Together, his attention to the future, his focus on the effectiveness of a "control program," and his emphasis on a targeted approach to a particular disease vector, anticipate aspects of techno-optimistic storytelling that would pervade later global health efforts.

CDC Is Born

Robert Woodruff's practical approach to malaria control in the southern United States was to become a significant factor in the federal government's decision about where to locate CDC. After the United States entered World War II in December 1941, enlisted soldiers were transported to newly constructed military camps in the American South, where the climate was better for year-round training. Many fell ill with malaria (Andrews 1946: 1).[11] During the war, combating malaria thus became a national security issue. In response, the US Public Health Service (USPHS) established the Office of Malaria Control in War Areas (MCWA) in 1942 in Atlanta.[12] In addition to its proximity to malaria-infested areas and its status as a transportation hub for the south, one reason USPHS chose Atlanta rather than Washington, DC was a "lack of space in Washington due to the war effort."[13] Woodruff's earlier funding of anti-malaria efforts also meant that there was a cadre of doctors and other public health professionals in Atlanta who were experts in malaria control. This established the city as a center of expertise on the disease.

When MCWA was established in Atlanta in 1942,

> The first offices were modest, just three or four rooms and a bay on the sixth floor of the Volunteer building on Peachtree Street, but it was enough for the small, sophisticated staff. Although the [public health department] provided most of the leadership, people were recruited from academe, other federal agencies, and wherever expertise about malaria existed. This expertise was in short supply.
>
> (Etheridge 1992: 4)

After the conclusion of World War II in 1946, MCWA was converted into the CDC with headquarters in downtown Atlanta and a laboratory division in Chamblee, a north-eastern suburb of the city (Carlisle 2020).

The next year, Robert Woodruff made a deal with Emory leaders that resulted in the university selling land to build new offices for CDC near the university for the sum of ten dollars. However, much of CDC operations would not move to the Emory campus until later in the 1950s after Woodruff called his friend—President Eisenhower—on the phone and demanded that congress fund its construction.

Though not mentioned in any histories, there was also a notable overlap between Woodruff's support for CDC in the 1940s and the expansion of Coca-Cola into international markets during World War II. In what has been celebrated as a smart marketing move, during the war Robert Woodruff promoted Coca-Cola as a drink for the military abroad and offered it at a discounted cost of five cents per bottle. The US government took Woodruff up on his offer, financed most of the transport costs for the beverage, and paid much of the cost for parts needed to build new bottling plants where troops were stationed around the world (sixty-four were in operation by the end of the war) (Barnes 1985).[14] And Woodruff became a prominent and influential advocate for CDC after the end of the war. This presages the intertwining of international business, government, education, and philanthropy that was to become a common feature of global health.

The Role of Novel Technologies in CDC's Origin Story

It is unclear how long-lived MCWA might have been were it not for the development of dichloro-diphenyl-trichloroethane (DDT)—the first modern synthetic insecticide—in the early 1940s.[15] DDT was regulated in the 1950s and 1960s and then banned in 1972 by the Environmental Protection Agency (EPA) after it became known that it was a carcinogen with harmful effects on animal (including human) reproduction. Before that time, however, it was widely used. A GHC video recorded in 1986 titled "CDC 40 years of prevention" features an interview segment about DDT and MCWA with Dr. Harry D. Pratt, an entomologist and one of the earliest members of MCWA and CDC.[16] In the video, Pratt tells a story about his earliest experiences working in public health, including the discovery of DDT:

Excerpt 2: The New Wonder Insecticide

FROM CDC 40 YEARS OF PREVENTION, 1 MIN 03 SEC

> Pratt: I went to Puerto Rico in 1942 to work on malaria control with the Insular Health Department. We made a fundamental decision that the MCWA, the Malaria Control in War Areas Program, would work around military bases and the Insular Health Department would

> continue to work in the cities. At the beginning of the program we used Paris Green[17] and oil on the waters and then we did a tremendous amount of drainage of malaria mosquito breeding places. In the Fall of 1944 an entomologist came down from the technical development laboratory in Savannah, Georgia, and brought with him samples of the new wonder insecticide DDT.

Pratt continues his story, explaining a test that his group conducted by comparing malaria in two Puerto Rican villages, one sprayed with DDT and the other not. Infection rates were dramatically lower in the village that had been sprayed. Pratt says, "so we felt that this was a wonderful deal," going on to talk about the DDT spraying program in the United States from 1945 to 1952. He concludes (at 2 min 41 sec), "We think that these DDT residual sprayings along with new drugs like Aderdrin and Primaquine plus very careful case histories led to the eradication of malaria from the United States and Puerto Rico."

Since this story is about the past rather than the future, it cannot properly be described as optimistic. However, Pratt's emphasis on DDT as a technological hero certainly matches techno-optimism in other ways. Focusing on actions taken, Pratt begins by narrating his experiences in the simple past tense ("I went," and "we made"). The temporal structure of the story becomes more complicated when Pratt uses the prepositional phrase, "at the beginning of the program," indicating a forward-looking attention to some sort of a change or shift that might occur. Pratt discusses the use of oil (floating on the top of water to discourage mosquito breeding) and the insecticide Paris green. Then he marks a turning point: a "new wonder insecticide," DDT. He also provides an epistemic claim on behalf of the field, "we think" that it was new technologies (DDT, Aderdrin, and Primaquine) alongside case histories that eradicated malaria from the United States and Puerto Rico. Pratt uses these linguistic markers and plot building blocks to construct a story about how new technology greatly improved human health in a manner that could be generalized to other communities and places.

On the question of whether or not this story is actually accurate: some scholars do not agree that new technologies played the pivotal role in malaria eradication efforts. It is true that after this and other experimental insecticide trials, including a successful intervention near Rome, Italy, international health experts made the determination that DDT spraying was the key to malaria control. However, "this conclusion ignored other factors that contributed to the success of this campaign," including decades of previous malaria-control efforts (Packard 2016: 107–108). Many years of previous public health efforts meant that "[the inhabitants of the region] were both informed about the disease and responsive to control efforts."

In addition, "the campaign itself generated widespread employment, which may have contributed to an overall improvement in health" (Packard 2016: 107–108). In other words, cultural and socioeconomic factors played an important role in the success of the Italian anti-malaria intervention. Significantly, a CDC Bulletin from 1946 mentions community education programs as important in its malaria eradication efforts (Andrews 1946: 1). The MCWA interventions were also enacted with populations who had little or no say in the matter (among military recruits and in a US territory). Despite all this, the narrative told by a public health elder (Pratt) forty years later emphasizes novel technologies as the heroes of the campaign. In this public health origin story, attention to socioeconomic inequities and structural changes was pushed aside in favor of the idea of reliance on simple technological fixes.

1950s–1970s: WHO, Communism, Civil Rights, and Smallpox Eradication

The MCWA technically became obsolete after the conclusion of World War II. However, the program had established a method and structure for coordination among various state health departments and USPHS, while also amassing a number of experts in the field of "exotic" and zoonotic diseases.[18] This led the US government to convert the MCWA into the Communicable Disease Center in 1946. At that time, the transformation was justified in the following ways:

> (1) as a safeguard against a recurrence of that unfortunate state of affairs which prevailed in 1942, when this nation could not find enough competent malaria control teams to service the Army and Navy overseas and to protect the health of its civilians at home; (2) as a prevention against the establishment of exotic infections introduced into this country by returning veterans, occupational troops, or as a result of constantly increasing global air traffic; and (3) to combat certain endemic infections… which are progressively infiltrating and entrenching themselves in new sections of the United States.
>
> (Andrews 1946: 4–5)

As this list indicates, much of the early justification for CDC's existence centered on the military and on the targeted neutralization of external threats posed by diseases from elsewhere—especially from the tropics. This health security justification remains a key part of contemporary global health storytelling, especially in the service of securing government funding (Lakoff 2010).

While the nascent CDC was outward-facing (searching for threats coming from outside the borders of the United States), the institution was to become focused on the health of Americans. It would be another new post-World War II institution that would organize international health efforts: the World Health Organization (WHO). WHO had a number of key antecedents and influences, including the International Sanitary Office of the American Republics (est. 1902, later became the Pan American Sanitary Bureau then the Pan American Health Organization), the Rockefeller Foundation (especially its International Health Division), the European-based Office Internationale d'Hygiène Publique (est. 1907 in Paris), and the League of Nations Health Organization (est. 1920 in Geneva) (Brown, Cueeto, and Fee 2006: 64). The United Nations (UN) replaced the League of Nations as part of a shift in the international balance of power in the wake of World War II, with Germany defeated and the United States and the USSR (the Union of Soviet Socialist Republics or Soviet Union, the bulk of which is now Russia) positioning themselves as new global powers.

WHO was established to provide a complement to the UN in the realm of health and sanitation. Here, there was a notable continuity with earlier colonial health efforts (Greene et al. 2013). Indeed, the key players, methods, and strategies remained largely the same:

> As before, [interventions] were designed by experts who met in cities in Europe and the United States to discuss and make plans for improving the health of peoples living in Africa, Asia, and Latin America. They also shared a confidence in the superiority of Western knowledge and a disregard both for the ideas and practices of those for whom the campaigns were created and for the ability of targeted populations to meet their own health needs. They also paid little attention to the underlying social and economic determinants of health or the need to develop basic health services.
>
> (Packard 2016: 90)

Though the development of WHO is fascinating and important, it is largely outside the scope of this chapter's focus on Atlanta (see Packard 2016 for more on the history of WHO; Brown, Cueeto, and Fee 2006). However, the continuation of this pattern—of interventions crafted in high-income countries (former colonizers) for the benefit of low-income countries (former colonized peoples)—is important to note, as it is an important criticism being made by contemporary scholars and practitioners who wish to decolonize global health.

The Atlanta-based CDC's early involvement with WHO was limited, regulated as it was by its official focus on health in the United States and

US territories. However, by the late 1940s American policy was rapidly becoming outward-facing as the country competed with the Soviet Union to establish world dominance in the ongoing contest that became known as the cold war. In 1949, in his second inaugural address, President Truman provided four foreign policy goals, the fourth of which was to "embark on a bold new program for making the benefits of our scientific advances and industrial progress available for the improvement and growth of underdeveloped areas."[19] After this policy shift, foreign public health specialists increasingly visited CDC for training—for instance, over 400 specialists from 66 countries visited in 1950 (Etheridge 1992: 24).

WHO launched its Malaria Eradication Program (MEP) in 1955. At the start, the United States provided funding and expertise but was not directly in charge. In 1966, however, CDC took control of the program. Available sources do not provide any clarity as to what prompted this shift, though there is a correlation between this takeover and the United States' official entrance into the Vietnam War in 1965 (Etheridge 1992: 179). Up to that point, the MEP had been largely successful. Still, it was becoming clear to some of the world's experts that eradication was likely impossible. For instance,

> Dr. Justin Andrews, CDC's former chief and one of the world's experts on malaria, had doubts. He knew it was technically feasible to eliminate malaria in spite of insecticide-resistant mosquitoes and drug-resistant strains. What concerned him were "resistances" from administrative, educational, and financial sources. He thought that WHO and [the Agency for International Development] should seek advice from the most knowledgeable authorities in the social sciences as to how these "resistances" might be overcome. Andrews proved to be a prophet.
>
> (Etheridge 1992: 180)

While this advocacy of social sciences by former CDC chief Andrews is laudable, his description of cultural and structural patterns as "resistances" mirrors the problematic "culture as barrier" model described in the introduction to this book—a model that still pervades much of public and global health. Indeed, knowledgeable authorities (at least in anthropology) would suggest that effective health interventions must be built "from the ground up," involving communities, governments, and health professionals of target populations meaningfully in decision-making, design, and implementation from the very beginning of a project. In conjunction with the fact that malaria control occurred primarily through pesticides (to which *anopheles* mosquitoes could become resistant) rather than through a vaccine, the challenges associated with not building malaria interventions from the ground up meant that malaria was never eradicated, though some regions of the world (such as the US South) were deemed malaria-free. For disease eradication, the world would have to wait for the Smallpox Eradication Program.

A Brief Note on Terminology: From Third World to Global South

The cold war would continue to shape global health until after the dissolution of the Soviet Union in 1991. One enduring impact of the conflict is the terminology used by global health professionals, social scientists, and the public to refer to regions of the world defined by socioeconomics and politics. In the early 1950s, some social scientists divided the globe into three "worlds": the first world, comprising the United States, Western Europe, and allied capitalist countries; the second "world," comprising the Soviet Union and its communist allies; and the third "world," those countries allied with neither the capitalists nor the communists. By the 1990s, with the threat of communist expansion neutralized, the "second world" term all but disappeared. Meanwhile, "third world" would begin to be replaced by capitalist terms: undeveloped, underdeveloped, and, later, developing. Most recently, the concept of the global South has become popular, using a spatial metaphor to indicate the significance of the history of power and colonialism in shaping contemporary international inequities.

None of these terms are truly up to the task of accurately modeling the complexities of wealth and power dynamics around the globe. "Third world" is a relic of the cold war and is often associated with negative stereotypes rooted in racism. "Undeveloped" ignores the history of colonialism and imperialism by which the countries in question came to be in such an unequal relationship with former colonizers (Rodney 1972). Underdeveloped (which frames a lack of development as the result of colonialism) and developing are better, but both are mired in capitalist ideologies and tend to assume a trajectory of progress toward Euro-American models of what it means to be a "developed" country. If one must use a term, I think global South is perhaps best (as can be seen in the title of this book). The concept of global South begins with the fact that most low-income, formerly colonized countries are located in the southern hemisphere and provides an analysis of economic and power differentials between countries of the "global South" and the "global North." However, I tend to also avoid this term when possible because it has the effect of reducing attention of the role and significance of inequities internal to both the global South and the global North in maintaining global hierarchies. When necessary, I often simply use the UN classification of low-income, middle-income, and high-income countries, which have the benefit of being tied to something measurable, if problematically so (gross domestic product [GDP]).[20]

The Civil Rights Movement, Public Health, and the USPHS Syphilis Study

As mentioned, CDC was relatively inactive internationally in the 1950s and early 1960s, though it was involved in the training of foreign health professionals. In the United States itself, in 1957 the Venereal Disease Division of USPHS was transferred to CDC. This doubled CDC's budget and also brought the administration of a program that was to become infamous—the USPHS Syphilis Study at Tuskegee—to Atlanta (Etheridge 1992: 87–91). The USPHS Syphilis Study was only a small part of the Venereal Disease Division and was outside of the purview of CDC for the first twenty-five years of the study's duration, but it is significant that CDC did not stop the study even after questions about its ethics began to be raised internally. The study is also important to consider because it has had a large impact on public health, social science, and global health discourses about race, inequities, research, and health care (Reverby 2009: 228). Revelations about the unethical nature of the Syphilis Study were significant in the US government's creation of the Belmont Report in 1979,[21] which has shaped national laws and policies for the protection of human subjects in biomedical and behavior research ever since (Hussein and Upshur 2013: 105). And variations on these laws and policies have been exported to other countries around the world as institutional review boards proliferate in low- and middle-income countries and health professionals in those countries attempt to reduce the exploitation of low-income populations in international medical studies.

The USPHS Syphilis Study was initiated long before civil rights would become a keyword in mainstream discourses, though it commenced after the beginning of the struggle for civil rights in the United States. Initiated in 1932 in Tuskegee, Alabama, the Syphilis Study was a research project designed to document the progression of untreated syphilis. Without fully explaining the study and without obtaining what is now known as "informed consent" to participate, 600 Black men were enrolled—399 with syphilis and 201 who were not infected. Individuals were enticed into the study by offering them benefits that were unheard of among Black Americans at that time, especially in the South: "medical exams, rides to and from the clinics, meals on examination days, free treatment for minor ailments and guarantees that provisions would be made after their deaths in terms of burial stipends paid to their survivors."[22] According to CDC's contemporary description of the study, "Researchers told the men they were being treated for 'bad blood,' a local term used to describe several ailments, including syphilis, anemia, and fatigue."[23] Both infected and non-infected individuals were given aspirin and iron tonic, with doctors implying that these were treatments for bad blood though this was not the case—the "treatment" was a placebo (Reverby 2009: 1). By the mid-1940s, penicillin became well-known among doctors as an effective treatment for syphilis, but study participants were still not treated with penicillin nor told about this development.[24] It was not until 1972 that Jean Heller of the associated press published a report in multiple newspapers lambasting the study's withholding of treatment for forty years. Public outcry then pushed the Assistant Secretary for Health and Scientific Affairs to create a panel to review the project. The panel ultimately described the study as "ethically unjustified," and in 1973 study participants and their families filed a successful class-action suit, resulting in a settlement of over nine million dollars.[25]

Much has been written about the unethical nature of the USPHS Syphilis Study. Critiques include: failure to inform potential participants about the true nature of the study and thus failure to obtain consent; use of outsized economic incentives to coerce participation; and failure to treat all infected individuals and stop the study when it became clear that penicillin was a cure for syphilis. These actions and non-actions provide plot points for powerful contemporary stories about racism and medicine:

> The symbolic power of "Tuskegee" works because of the revulsion over the idea that the PHS deceived men and their families, waited for years as they died, whether from syphilis or not, and then carved up their bodies at autopsies.
>
> (Reverby 2009: 232)

The USPHS Syphilis Study was not the first or the only example of unethical medical research, but it is one of the most well-known. During the COVID-19 pandemic, the study was often cited in discussions about why Black Americans were hesitant to be vaccinated. However, the study's significance is sometimes overemphasized. Distrust of the medical establishment is rooted in a much longer history of medical abuse of Black persons and contemporary experiences of medical racism (Washington 2006; Carter 2022).[26]

An additional significance of the Syphilis Study is what can be learned from it about CDC's approach to civil rights in the 1960s. Especially with CDC's location in an important civil rights city, some employees were active in the civil rights movement. In addition, CDC leaders were quietly pushing for more professional parity and protection of rights inside the organization (Etheridge 1992: 118–119). Within the cultural context of the time period, which included rampant overt racism and disregard for the health and well-being of people of color, CDC's "color-blind" application of scientific medicine to all and its efforts to treat diseases that disproportionately affected BIPOC (Black, Indigenous, and People of Color) communities in the United States and abroad were arguably evidence of an anti-racist approach. In terms of official efforts, however, the institution seems to have had no involvement at all in civil rights discourses. Nothing related to civil rights is mentioned on the CDC museum's website[27]; and the Venereal Disease Division has (understandably, in the context of the Syphilis Study) been described in published work as "insensitive to the civil rights movement" (Etheridge 1992: 91). This noticeable absence of public-facing civil rights initiatives and CDC's inaction in response to the USPHS Syphilis Study—despite the internal efforts of CDC leaders—provides an indication of how dominant discourses and politics may shape and limit government-based public health institutions. In other words, CDC was (and is) a government institution and could not take a public stance on a movement as controversial as the civil rights movement was at the time without attracting the ire of the politicians that funded the institution. As will be discussed in the next chapter, the inability to avoid the whims of the political moment in public institutions is one reason some global health professionals prefer what they call "public-private partnerships."

Bill Foege's Story about the Smallpox Eradication Program

Not long before the USPHS Syphilis Study became notorious, WHO was also ramping up the Smallpox Eradication Program (SEP). This program was first devised in the early 1950s and then reintroduced as a WHO proposal by the Soviet Union in 1958. Surprisingly, given the Soviet Union's spearheading of the movement, the United States also supported smallpox eradication efforts. However, the United States focused its support specifically in West Africa. The idea behind this targeted support was that smallpox eradication could be a way to exert political influence through humanitarian work at a time when many African nations were gaining independence and thus could potentially be swayed toward communism by the Soviet Union.

There were several characteristics of the smallpox virus and its treatment that made smallpox eradication more likely than malaria eradication: (1) it was a pathogen that was transmitted from human to human via airborne droplets of saliva (without an animal intermediary, as with malaria); (2) the illness had clear symptoms and no asymptomatic transmission; (3) there was a vaccine that had been proven to be effective; and (4) there was a newly discovered method of freeze-drying vaccines to enable them to be transported to and administered in warm climates. However, the campaign was not truly within reach of succeeding until it was discovered that targeted surveillance, containment, and vaccination of outbreaks could work effectively (as opposed to mass vaccinations, which were economically and practically untenable) (Packard 2016: 144–145, 164).

Dr. William Foege, introduced at the beginning of this chapter, was a key player in this discovery and a hero of the SEP—especially in some of the stories told by Atlanta-area global health professionals. After finishing his medical degree at the age of twenty-six, Foege worked as an Epidemic Intelligence Service (EIS) Officer for CDC in Colorado from 1962 to 1964. He then attended the Harvard School of Public Health to earn a Master of Public Health degree in 1965.[28] While working as an EIS officer, CDC sent him overseas twice—first to India, and then to Tonga, where he helped study how much the smallpox vaccine could be diluted and still be effective.

The GHC has a large collection of Foege-related archival materials. Among these is an interview conducted by Victoria Harden in 2006 about Foege's early life and experiences with SEP.[29] Foege would later publish his account in a book on the subject of smallpox eradication (Foege 2012). His extended story is fascinating, providing a window into life as an expat in low-income countries in the 1960s. This lifestyle was broadly similar to that of anthropologists who worked in the same areas at that time.[30] Indeed, Foege portrays himself as somewhat of a swashbuckling figure. For instance, he returned to Nigeria in the midst of a civil war after being arrested, deported, and told not to return (but, he says, they were not keeping good records at the time, so he was not too worried about being discovered).

In the GHC interview, Foege explains that after graduating from Harvard, where he had in fact done an academic project on smallpox eradication, he took a position with a Christian medical commission through the World Council of Churches. He then moved with his family to Nigeria to promote community medicine with that group. Soon after, though, CDC asked him if he would be a consultant for SEP, so Foege traveled to Atlanta in 1966 to take a summer course designed for people working on SEP in Africa.

In Foege's telling, the big breakthrough for SEP came on the eve of the Nigerian civil war. In the interview (p. 10–11 of the transcript), Harden asks about the approach that Foege had taken in his Harvard class project about smallpox eradication. Foege replies, "Everyone in those days was thinking in terms of mass vaccination." At that time, it was thought that the only viable strategy for eliminating smallpox from a population was to vaccinate the vast majority of people.

But then Foege describes the beginnings of an outbreak in Ogoga province, Nigeria, and his efforts to diagnose the illness. He continues,

Excerpt 3: Foege Smallpox Eradication, Part 1

GHC TRANSCRIPT PAGE 11

> Foege: It was so early in the program, we didn't have much in the way of supplies, and then I learned we wouldn't get any more supplies. We were faced with the question of how to use our small amount of smallpox vaccine most effectively under these conditions. That night, we went to

> a missionary's house to take advantage of the fact that they got on the radio with each other at 7pm each night to be sure no one was having a medical emergency. With maps in front of me, I was able to give each missionary a geographic area and ask if they could send runners to every village in that area to find out if there were any smallpox cases in any of the villages. Twenty-four hours later, we got back on the radio to see what they had found. That night we knew exactly where smallpox was. Our strategy was to use most of the vaccine in the villages where we knew that smallpox existed.

In this story's construction, it is significant that in the second sentence Foege pauses his chronological recounting of events. He does so in order to summarize, "We were faced with the question of how to use our small amount of smallpox vaccine most effectively under these conditions." This frames the story as linked to a core ethical value in contemporary global health: using available (limited) resources most effectively (see Chapter 3).

Foege then describes his small group's decision-making process about how to allocate the tiny remaining amount of vaccine:

Excerpt 4: Foege Smallpox Eradication, Part 2

GHC TRANSCRIPT PAGE 11

> Foege: we tried to out-figure the smallpox virus. I mean, we literally asked ourselves, "If we were a smallpox virus bent on immortality, what would we do?" The answer was to find susceptible hosts in order to continue growing. So we figured out where people were likely to go because of market patterns and family patterns. We chose three areas that we thought were susceptible, and we used the rest of our vaccine to vaccinate those three areas. That used up all of our vaccine. We didn't know it, but in two of the areas, smallpox was already incubating, but by the time the first clinical cases appeared, those areas had been vaccinated. And so smallpox went no place. By three or four weeks later, the outbreak had stopped. And we had vaccinated such a small proportion of the population!

With this exclamation Foege ends this part of his story. The efficiency of the method that Foege and his colleagues developed was indeed notable. It made eradication "cost-effective," meaning it did not require a large infusion of money that political and business leaders were unwilling to provide.

Later in the interview, Foege compares his effort with another effort in a different region where the group had used the broad vaccination approach, noting that targeted vaccinations alongside surveillance actually worked better. The interviewer (Harden) summarizes, "So you knew by then that this method of 'surveillance/containment' or 'eradication escalation'—whatever term we are going to use—was a more effective way to eradicate smallpox" (13). The Nigerian civil war soon interrupted Foege's work and he ended up back at CDC. In fact, it was not until several years later that the team was able to go back to Nigeria and determine that their program had truly halted smallpox's progress in the region. After that, it then took a number of years to get other SEP country/regional programs to agree to shift to this targeted model, but most did, and smallpox was officially declared eradicated in 1980.

This is the only example of successful human disease eradication in recorded history; yet rather than describing smallpox eradication like an outlier or a non-repeatable event, many in the field of global health treat the story as an archetypal or mythical target for future interventions. Classic scholarship on narrative argues, "to be worth telling, a tale must be about how an implicit canonical script has been breached, violated, or deviated from" (Bruner 1991: 11). The canonical script that is breached in the smallpox story is the idea that mass vaccination (and in general, massive, generalized health interventions) is the only way to eradicate a disease. The new alternative is a targeted health campaign using limited resources efficiently through data-driven analysis and intervention.

Through this canonical breach, global health professionals present the smallpox eradication story as a reason for continuing to promote techno-optimistic visions of the eradication of other diseases. The idea of the epidemiologist with maps and phones directing the flow of health-care workers and medications also clearly resonates with contemporary white-collar approaches in the field. Recall that a neighbor who works in global health fundraising once told me that the unsung hero of smallpox eradication was a "guy in an office with a computer and a phone" directing the whole endeavor (though I am not sure how much CDC employees in the 1970s actually used computers). Regardless of the truth of this statement, it indicates that for some health professionals, the takeaway points from Bill Foege's story include that it is better to work smarter, that it is better for health care to be more technocratic, and that vaccines work.

1980s–2000s: Neoliberalism and the Rise of NPOs

In 1977, President Jimmy Carter chose Bill Foege to become director of the CDC, a role that Foege would hold until 1983, well into Ronald Reagan's presidency. During his time as director, Foege led the bureaucratic transition of the CDC from an agency that focused primarily on infectious diseases to one that oversaw public health in a broader sense, including non-communicable diseases, population health, and environmental health (Lane 2012). Throughout the 1960s and 1970s, the CDC consolidated a number of governmental health programs into the organization, including the tuberculosis program, immunization practices, nutrition, the National Institute for Occupational Safety and Health, and the Foreign Quarantine Service.[31] In recognition of its broadening scope of work, in 1970 the Communicable Disease Center was renamed the Center for Disease Control; and after Foege's reorganization in 1981, Center was pluralized to become "Centers" (Lane 2012).

After Ronald Reagan became president in 1981, Foege had to adapt to the president's aggressive neoliberalization efforts. This included massive budget cuts for the CDC and other government health agencies and deregulation of a wide swath of departments (e.g., reducing the Department of Agriculture's oversight of meat and poultry processing plants, rejecting a plan to require airbags in automobiles). This was the beginning of a worldwide push spearheaded by Reagan and his British counterpart, Prime Minister Margaret Thatcher, to privatize a range of fields including health care and public health (Terris 1999). One reason that they were able to consolidate political will for this effort was that the world was in the midst of a global recession catalyzed by the Iranian revolution and its impact on oil prices (a revolution that was itself tied to CIA interventions into Iranian politics earlier in the cold war).

Unfortunately for the health of much of the world's population, the global recession of the early 1980s came at around the same time that health leaders from the Soviet Union and other Communist countries were mobilizing to push WHO to support primary health care for all (called the "primary healthcare movement"). In the context of the recession, the policy idea of providing basic primary health care to all people regardless of ability to pay was quickly dismissed by many. Faced with reductions in health spending, the primary healthcare movement was soon replaced by a push for "*selective* primary health care" (for a detailed overview of this historical moment, see Basilico et al. 2013; Packard 2016: ch. 13). Selective primary health care revolved around "cost-effectiveness," which would develop into the ethical value of effectiveness in global health (see Chapter 3). The idea of GOBI is associated with this approach. GOBI, which is primarily focused on children and mothers, stands for growth monitoring, oral rehydration therapy (for treating diarrheal diseases), breastfeeding, and immunizations (Basilico et al. 2013: 82). One of the key organizations to support GOBI initiatives would be the Task Force for Child Survival (led by Bill Foege—see below).

One major organization that enthusiastically supported the selective primary healthcare movement was the World Bank. This was not surprising, given that the World Bank—with the International Monetary Fund (IMF) and in alignment with Reagan and Thatcher—had adopted structural adjustment policies. In the post-colonial political and economic turmoil that followed after African and Latin American nations declared independence from colonial powers in the 1960s and 1970s and struggled with being caught in between the political machinations of the United States and the USSR, many low-income countries' governments (sometimes run by autocratic rulers) took significant "loans" from the World Bank and IMF.[32] In order to qualify for further loans, it was decided that countries would be required to promote free market policies, reduce governmental programs, and denationalize various sectors of their economies. In this context, socialized government-run healthcare systems around the world were privatized to differing degrees or just not developed as many might have wished. Selective primary health care fit well with this trend toward limited healthcare provisioning.

Structural adjustment programs of the 1980s and 1990s left large gaps in care for the most marginalized, and NPOs proliferated to fill these gaps. These organizations were sometimes funded by the philanthropic efforts of the very same companies and CEOs who were directly benefiting from privatization and capital-fueled privatization. The rise of NPOs entailed new forms of governmentality and arrangements of power, as low- and middle-income nations without strong governments had a limited ability to control what NPOs based in high-income countries could or could not do (Fisher 1997; Ferguson and Gupta 2002). This was disastrous for the health of residents of low- and middle-income countries. Indeed, Jim Yong Kim—the global health expert who would be World Bank president from 2012 to 2019—and his colleagues condemned structural adjustment programs in the strongest terms, describing the world's poor as "dying for growth" (Kim et al. 2000).[33] The long-term impact of these development policies on public and global health has been profoundly negative (Pfeiffer and Chapman 2010). Many global health NPOs were formed in an attempt to address this problem.

Two Atlanta NPOs Are Born

It was in this geo-political context that two of the major Atlanta-area global health NPOs—the Task Force and the Carter Center—were founded, and Bill Foege played a key role in both. In early 1984 (the year after he left CDC), Foege and two of his former CDC colleagues created the Task Force for Child Survival. At that time, the newly formed Task Force facilitated a meeting in Italy that was organized by the Rockefeller Foundation and attended by the United Nations International Children's Emergency Fund (UNICEF). It was at that meeting that the previously mentioned GOBI approach to selective primary health care was developed (Foege 2018: 5).

This effort, which became known as the Child-Survival Revolution, was shaped by the priorities of "a group of predominantly white European and American public-health leaders, nearly all of whom were men," whose perspectives were rooted in "a vision of international health built on the provision of effective medical technologies to prevent and eventually eliminate diseases" (Packard 2016: 265). With these critiques in mind, though, it is important to note that with Bill Foege at the helm and the WHO and UNICEF on board, the Child-Survival Revolution (utilizing the GOBI approach) was indeed effective in greatly reducing child mortality in low-income countries by 1990.

In a book he wrote about the Task Force's early years, Foege touts the NPO's efforts as "the story of how successful coalitions happen" (Foege 2018: 6). Indeed, the Task Force pioneered the approaches that would become theorized as collaboration and public-private partnerships (more on this in Chapter 3). Still, the contrast between Foege's evaluation of the GOBI program and the perspective of a global health anthropologist critic is striking: "Within this environment, hopes of building primary health-care systems, let alone addressing the underlying social determinants of health... did not stand a chance. Neoliberal policies continued to shape global-health strategies into the twenty-first century" (Packard 2016: 264). As will be discussed in Chapter 3, the response of Bill Foege and many other contemporary global health professionals to such a critique was a pragmatic one: they did what they could with the resources at hand in the socioeconomic and political context in which they were operating.

Indeed, on multiple occasions Foege has emphasized that public health is fundamentally linked to politics; and he has said that this was especially so in the 1970s and 1980s when most funding for health initiatives came from governments. For instance, in one of his GHC interviews,[34] while talking about the Smallpox Eradication Campaign and his time as CDC director, Foege explains:

Excerpt 5: Foege Politics and Public Health (17 min 18 sec)

> Foege: Political problems can ruin your day, and yet every public health decision is based on a political decision. And if I have regrets, and I do, one of them is that I didn't learn how to operate politically early enough. Because public health people tend to think if we do the right thing, everyone is going to understand and they'll support it and they'll fund it. You have to learn how to deal with politicians and give them satisfaction in achieving the outcome of a coalition. They are a part of the coalition, and we're totally dependent in public health on appropriations from politicians.

In global health, however, the financial dependency on political appropriations was soon to be partially replaced dependence on philanthropy. In Atlanta, at least, this shift was in no small part due to Foege's initiatives—first with the Task Force, then the Carter Center, and finally in his work with Bill Gates.

A second key Atlanta-area global health NPO to be established in the 1980s was the Carter Center. The Carter Center, which is affiliated with Emory University, is an outgrowth of Jimmy Carter's presidential library established after the end of his presidency in 1981. It took a few years for the center itself to take shape, and it was not until 1986 that Bill Foege was appointed executive director and fellow for health policy for the center. Foege's appointment was part of Jimmy Carter's increasing interest in health interventions in low-income nations and communities.[35] According to the center's 1982–1988 report, the Task Force for Child Survival was integrated into the Carter Center during that time period, though the report does not say when this happened (perhaps when Foege became executive director).[36] For a time, then, the Task Force and Carter Center were two parts of the same organization, and to all appearances they continue to have a good working relationship in the present day.

Over the years, the Carter Center has led a number of international health initiatives, including a recent push to destigmatize global mental health care prompted by former first lady Rosalynn Carter's interests, but one of the center's most notable efforts has been the Guinea Worm Eradication Program started in 1986 under Foege's direction. This was after CDC started a global campaign to eradicate guinea worm disease in 1980 (when Foege was director of CDC).[37] According to the Carter Center's website,

> Guinea worm disease *could* become the second human disease in history, after smallpox, to be eradicated. It *would* be the first parasitic disease to be eradicated and the first disease to be eradicated without the use of a vaccine or medicine.
>
> (emphasis added)[38]

Unlike the SEP, the lack of a vaccine or medicine for guinea worm necessitates an approach that is not fully reliant on technology. Notably, though, the Carter Center does not advocate for structural change—at least not in public-facing discourse. Guinea worm disease "is transmitted by drinking water from ponds and other stagnant surface water sources" and "affects poor communities in remote parts of Africa that do not have safe water to drink."[39] The simplest solution—though a very expensive one—would be to build water treatment plants and infrastructure for water distribution. Yet the Carter Center focuses on education, "teaching people to filter all drinking water and preventing transmission by keeping anyone with an emerging worm from entering water sources."[40] The center's 1982–1988 report says that the organization was working to improve water supplies "and/or teach people to simply filter or boil their water."[41] However, as with many other health interventions, a focus on individual behavior ignores the very real structural constraints (aka the "social determinants of health") that prevent individuals from enacting behavioral changes. For instance, filtration and boiling require filters or fuel, either of which may seem to cost little to global health professionals and donors but may cost more than impoverished individuals can afford.

From its inception, the Carter Center was funded by donations made by individuals, foundations, and corporations, as well as the Carters themselves.[42] This means that it—along with the Task Force that was associated with it—was one of the first Atlanta-area secular global health NPOs.[43] Amid the privatization efforts of the 1980s and the waning influence of the Soviet Union and thus of communist approaches to care, Bill Foege led the way toward a new configuration of science, politics, and economics in Atlanta in order to continue to address public health problems in low- and middle-income countries. In this new configuration, however, the Carter Center and the Task Force focused on targeted (and often, technologically based) interventions in order to be effective with the limited resources at their disposal.

Some More Recent History

The 1990s and 2000s were times of transition in terms of global health governance. Without the communist counterbalance previously provided by the Soviet Union, neoliberalization of health institutions continued unabated and NPOs claimed larger roles in health governance. Beyond Atlanta, growing awareness that HIV/AIDS was rapidly spreading to a pandemic stage prompted dramatic shifts in economic priorities in the field. In 1986, WHO created what would later become the Global Program on AIDS (GPA), and by 1990 the GPA was the largest single program in the history of WHO, with ninety million US dollars' worth of funding (Packard 2016: 279). This and other HIV/AIDS initiatives of the 1990s disrupted the top-down hierarchical structure that had been associated with the concept of international health (with WHO and UN at the top), and new constellations of interests and coordination across organizations began to take shape that would become known as "partnerships" and "collaboration" (Rosenberg et al. 2010: 24). Large increases in US government funding for HIV/AIDS interventions also began in 2003 with President George W. Bush's creation of the US President's Emergency Plan for AIDS Relief (PEPFAR). PEPFAR was unusual for the time period because it was bilateral aid—between the United States and recipient countries—rather than multilateral (through WHO or UN) or collaborative (through NPOs). And the Bill and Melinda Gates Foundation's arrival on the global health scene by the early 2000s further upended established funding patterns.

In Atlanta, 1992 saw the arrival of CARE (Cooperative for Assistance and Relief Everywhere), which relocated its headquarters from New York. The Robert Woodruff Foundation bought, remodeled, and donated a five-story building in downtown Atlanta, and Atlanta civic and business leaders offered to pay for part of CARE's relocating costs and to provide free and discounted legal, accounting, and travel services (Rabinovitz 1992).[44] CARE is an organization that was created to provide food to war-torn regions of Europe after the conclusion of World War II, and from that time until the 1990s the organization was primarily involved in direct aid. CARE distributed foodstuffs and other needed items, with a focus on the needs of women and girls that developed over the decades. In the 1980s, CARE seems to have benefited from a close relationship with Vice President George H. W. Bush and began to receive funding from the US Agency for International Development (USAID). Notably, the NPO states that in 1992, it saw its largest year of expansion following the collapse of the Soviet Union as it worked to address gaps in social services previously provided by communist governments in Eastern Europe and beyond. While direct aid remains a key part of the organization's work, in the 2000s CARE branched out into education, HIV/AIDS, and water and sanitation, with funding from USAID and the Bill and Melinda Gates Foundation in addition to other private donors.[45]

Bill Foege became a senior medical adviser for the Bill and Melinda Gates Foundation in 1999. This was a major event for both the field as a whole and global health in Atlanta more specifically. The new relationship between the two Bills heralded the shift in the financial model for global health away from government and bilateral/multilateral funding toward philanthropic funding. Over time, this solidified relationship led to a rise to even further prominence for the Task Force for Global Health in the Atlanta metropolitan region.

CDC Foundation and the Institutionalization of Public-Private Partnerships

Another significant addition to the Atlanta NPO world was the creation of the CDC Foundation. A CDC leader named Martha Katz played an important role in the start of the foundation. One report (based on an interview with Katz) states, "Over the years, many CDC directors dreamed of having a CDC Foundation to capitalize on private support."[46] Congress passed legislation in 1992 to allow for the creation of an "independent, nonprofit foundation to support CDC," and the foundation began operations in 1995.[47] In addition to CDC Foundation's global health orientation, CDC itself continues to maintain its own robust international connections. Established in 2010, the CDC Center for Global Health (CGH) works primarily with governmental agencies (e.g., ministries of health abroad) and multilateral organizations.[48] Still, the CDC Foundation seems to focus more on programs outside the United States than inside.[49] By creating the CDC Foundation, congress institutionalized the idea of public-private partnership that had been shaping international health since the beginnings of CDC.

In 2018, this institutionalized public/private partnership would become the source of a conspiracy theory promoted by the founder and chairperson of CrossFit, Greg Glassman. Glassman "became concerned… about allegations that The Coca-Cola Company and other soft drink makers had used donations to the CDC Foundation to influence the charity's work" (Mervis 2018).[50] Ostensibly, Glassman's worry was rooted in the fact that soft drinks are detrimental to a person's health, and he felt that the Coca-Cola company's donations might lead the CDC to more favorably evaluate industry-sponsored research about "big soda, big pharma, and the alcohol industry."[51] The political hoopla that ensued focused on the question of transparency—something that the CDC Foundation did in fact attend to in ways similar to other NPOs (a topic to be discussed in Chapter 4).

Glassman's complaint, which was (perhaps not coincidentally) a great way to publicize and promote CrossFit, seems to have been made in ignorance of the ninety-year history of Coca-Cola's involvement in CDC work (though perhaps this would only have fueled the narrative). While it is doubtlessly true that the presence of Coca-Cola and the Woodruff Foundation as donor audiences has shaped public health narratives, and thus priorities, in ways discussed throughout this book, the idea that there is a direct link between donations and skewing of expert evaluation of research in the CDC Foundation seems baseless. Still, the ensuing public discussion about questions of transparency and the links between industry and public health perhaps helped produce the sorts of discursive environment that contributed to the anti-vaccine and pro-hydroxychloroquine movements during the COVID-19 pandemic (to be discussed in Chapter 5).

Conclusion

From the origins of CDC in Atlanta onward, the roots of the epistemic, ethical, and economic values of contemporary global health were apparent. These included an epistemic emphasis on evidence, testing, and technological development and an ethical emphasis on effectiveness and collaboration, with a mixed record with respect to issues of race and equity. Later, the economic values of global health were developed when the neoliberal policies of the 1980s led health professionals to shift health governance toward increased reliance on NPOs and philanthropy.

Atlanta was perhaps not the most obvious candidate to become a global health hub. While it has long been a regional center for transportation, it is land-locked and far from the intellectual/philanthropic/governmental hubs of New York and Washington, DC; yet its location in a malaria-infested region, alongside the scholarly acumen offered by Emory University and the support of the philanthropically oriented leader of a company that was rapidly becoming successful on an international scale (Coca-Cola), helped Atlanta to find its place as a source of international health expertise. Most recently, Atlanta has become an international travel center—in fact, Atlanta's airport is now the busiest in the world. Having the world within reach by air travel has no doubt only reinforced the city's ability to operate as a global health hub. The Task Force for Global Health, the Carter Center, and Emory University have been joined by other universities and NPOs that often exchange personnel with CDC, such as the CDC Foundation, CARE, and several universities in the metropolitan region (including Georgia State University, whose school of public health was accredited in 2016). This mix of public, private, and philanthropic organizations makes health global in Atlanta.

Notes

1 https://www.youtube.com/watch?v=qgZwroXzar8&t=61s. Accessed 6/1/2023
2 This is a consortium comprising historically Black colleges and universities including Clark Atlanta University, Morehouse College, Morehouse School of Medicine, and Spelman College.
3 "Atlanta in 50 Objects: Robert W. Woodruff," https://www.atlantahistorycenter.com/exhibitions/atlanta-in-50-objects/robert-w-woodruff/. Accessed 3/13/2023.
4 http://whsc.emory.edu/about/history/timeline.html and https://www.cdc.gov/museum/app/roots/roots.html.
5 https://www.georgiawomen.org/copy-of-wilson-ellen-louise-axson. Accessed 3/13/2023; and https://findingaids.library.emory.edu/documents/woodruff47/printable/. Accessed 5/8/2023.
6 https://findingaids.library.emory.edu/documents/woodruff10/. Accessed 5/8/2023.
7 "Robert W. Woodruff Correspondence," *The Global Health Chronicles*, https://globalhealthchronicles.org/items/show/4682. Accessed 3/13/2023.
8 https://www.gghalliance.org/global-health-atl. Accessed 5/24/2023; in 2013 a steering committee was established that included the Task Force for Global Health, the National Health Museum, Morehouse School of Medicine, CARE, Emory University, the Carter Center, and the CDC Foundation.
9 "Dr. Melvin Goodwin," *The Global Health Chronicles*, p. 5, https://globalhealthchronicles.org/items/show/4679. Accessed 3/13/2023.
10 https://globalhealthchronicles.org/items/show/5051. Accessed 5/9/2023.

11 https://www.cdc.gov/museum/app/roots/roots.html. Accessed 3/2/2023. Please note that this and many other CDC webpages cited in this book have been removed by the current government administration.
12 https://globalhealthchronicles.org/malaria-beginnings. Accessed 3/9/2023.
13 https://www.washingtonpost.com/archive/local/1985/03/09/coca-cola-tycoon-robert-woodruff-dies-at-age-95/ef115e86–3258-4ce4-a4e2-cb161f475a60/. Accessed 5/8/2023.
14 https://www.epa.gov/ingredients-used-pesticide-products/ddt-brief-history-and-status. Accessed 3/3/2023.
15 https://globalhealthchronicles.org/items/show/5340. Accessed 3/9/2023.
16 Paris Green is a green powder with arsenic that was used as an insecticide.
17 I place the term "exotic" diseases in quotes because the definition of what counts as exotic (in other words, foreign) depends on the location from which one defines the term.
18 https://www.trumanlibrary.gov/sites/default/files/InternationalAid_Background.pdf. Accessed 5/10/2023.
19 https://www.npr.org/sections/goatsandsoda/2015/01/04/372684438/if-you-shouldnt-call-it-the-third-world-what-should-you-call-it. Accessed 9/4/24.
20 https://www.hhs.gov/ohrp/regulations-and-policy/belmont-report/read-the-belmont-report/index.html. Accessed 5/16/2023.
21 https://www.tuskegee.edu/about-us/centers-of-excellence/bioethics-center/about-the-usphs-syphilis-study. Accessed 5/17/2023.
22 https://www.cdc.gov/tuskegee/timeline.htm. Accessed 5/16/2023.
23 https://www.tuskegee.edu/about-us/centers-of-excellence/bioethics-center/about-the-usphs-syphilis-study. Accessed 5/16/2023.
24 https://www.tuskegee.edu/about-us/centers-of-excellence/bioethics-center/about-the-usphs-syphilis-study. Accessed 5/16/2023.
25 https://www.npr.org/2021/02/16/967011614/in-tuskegee-painful-history-shadows-efforts-to-vaccinate-african-americans. Accessed 5/15/2023; and https://www.npr.org/sections/health-shots/2021/03/23/974059870/stop-blaming-tuskegee-critics-say-its-not-an-excuse-for-current-medical-racism. Accessed 5/15/2023.
26 https://www.cdc.gov/museum/timeline/1940–1970.html#1950. Accessed 5/15/2023.
27 https://sph.emory.edu/departments/gh/fellows/foege/bill-foege/index.html. Accessed 5/12/2023.
28 https://globalhealthchronicles.org/items/show/3516. Accessed 5/12/2023.
29 A transcript of this interview can be found here: https://globalhealthchronicles.org/files/original/817185efe3d9b4f4fe6938e66252dcac.pdf.
30 "Historical Perspectives History of CDC" *Morbidity and Mortality Weekly Report*, June 28, 1996, https://www.cdc.gov/mmwr/preview/mmwrhtml/00042732.htm#:~:text=Finally%2C%20in%20October%201992%2C%20Congress,global%20leader%20in%20public%20health. Accessed 5/22/2023.
31 I put loans in quotations because the term "loan" is a misleading way to describe the process wherein wealth that had been violently extracted from colonized countries by colonial powers was then provided to those same countries, but with strings attached and a requirement to repay with interest.
32 Kim has an M.D., was trained as an anthropologist, and worked closely with M.D./anthropologist/global health leader Paul Farmer for over a decade to build the NPO "Partners in Health"

33 Foege, William H. interview by Dr. Bess Miller on August 26, 2016. *The Global Health Chronicles,* https://globalhealthchronicles.org/items/show/6480. Accessed 5/23/2023.
34 https://www.cartercenter.org/about/history/chronology_1981–1990.html. Accessed 5/22/2023; and https://sph.emory.edu/departments/gh/fellows/foege/bill-foege/index.html. Accessed 3/3/2023.
35 https://www.cartercenter.org/resources/pdfs/pdf-archive/annualreport1982–1988–01011989.pdf. p. 1. Accessed 5/23/2023.
36 https://www.cdc.gov/globalhealth/resources/reports/annual/2022/timeline.html. Accessed 9/7/23.
37 https://www.cartercenter.org/health/guinea_worm/index.html. Accessed 5/23/2023.
38 https://www.cdc.gov/parasites/guineaworm/index.html. Accessed 5/23/2023.
39 https://www.cartercenter.org/health/guinea_worm/index.html. Accessed 5/23/2023.
40 https://www.cartercenter.org/resources/pdfs/pdf-archive/annualreport1982–1988–01011989.pdf. p. 82 Accessed 5/23/2023.
41 https://www.cartercenter.org/resources/pdfs/pdf-archive/annualreport1982–1988–01011989.pdf pp. 92–97. Accessed 5/23/2023.
42 I say secular even though Jimmy and Rosalyn Carter have been vocal about the Christian motivations for their work, because the organization itself is not organized as a Christian organization.
43 https://www.nytimes.com/1992/09/20/nyregion/care-headquarters-to-move-to-atlanta-from-manhattan.html. Accessed 5/24/2023.
44 https://www.care.org/about-us/our-history/. Accessed 5/24/2023.
45 https://www.sophe.org/news/sophe-names-martha-katz-mpa-its-2022-honorary-fellow/and https://www.ianphi.org/_includes/documents/sections/tools-resources/best-practices-case-studies/foundation-bp-case-study_cdc-.pdf. Accessed 3/24/2023.
46 https://www.cdcfoundation.org/FAQ. Accessed 5/24/2023.
47 https://www.cdc.gov/globalhealth/resources/reports/annual/2022/cdc-75-years.html#:~:text=CDC%20established%20the%20Center%20for,emergency%20response%2C%20and%20workforce%20development. Accessed 8/7/2023.
48 see https://www.cdcfoundation.org/programs-list.
49 https://www.science.org/content/article/us-lawmakers-want-nih-and-cdc-foundations-say-more-about-donors. Accessed 5/30/2023.
50 https://www.prnewswire.com/news-releases/crossfit-inc-exposes-conflicts-of-interest-at-foundations-for-the-nih-and-cdc-300671847.html. Accessed 5/30/2023.

References

Andrews, Justin M. 1946. "Development of the Communicable Disease Center." In *The CDC Bulletin July, August, September 1946*, p. 1–12. Atlanta, GA: Federal Security Agency/ U.S. Public Health Service.

Barnes, Bart. 1985. "Coca-Cola Tycoon Robert Woodruff Dies at Age 95." *The Washington Post*, March 9, 1985. https://www.washingtonpost.com/archive/local/1985/03/09/coca-cola-tycoon-robert-woodruff-dies-at-age-95/ef115e86-3258-4ce4-a4e2-cb161f475a60/.

Basilico, Matthew, Jonathan Weigel, Anjali Motgi, Jacob Bor, and Salmaan Keshavjee. 2013. "Health For All? Competing Theories and Geopolitics." In *Reimagining Global Health: An Introduction*, edited by Paul Farmer, Jim Yong Kim, Arthur Kleinman, and Matthew Basilico, 74–110. Berkeley: University of California Press.

Brown, Theodore M., Marcos Cueeto, and Elizabeth Fee. 2006. "The World Health Organization and the Transition from International to Global Public Health." *American Journal of Public Health* 96: 62–72.

Bruner, Jerome. 1991. "The Narrative Construction of Reality." *Critical Inquiry* 18 (1): 1–21.

Carlisle, Lois. 2020. "For the Health of the Nation: A History of the CDC in Atlanta." Atlanta History Center. Accessed 3/2/2023.https://www.atlantahistorycenter.com/blog/a-history-of-the-cdc-in-atlanta/.

Carter, Chelsea. 2022. "Gaslighting: ALS, Anti-Blackness, and Medicine." *Feminist Anthropology* 3 (2): 181–411.

Etheridge, Elizabeth W. 1992. *Sentinel for Health: A History of the Centers for Disease Control*. Berkeley: University of California Press.

Ferguson, James, and Akhil Gupta. 2002. "Spatializing States: Toward an Ethnography of Neoliberal Governmentality." *American Ethnologist* 29 (4): 981–1002.

Fisher, William. 1997. "Doing Good? The Politics and Antipolitics of NGO Practices." *Annual Review of Anthropology* 26: 439–464.

Foege, William. 2012. *House on Fire: The Fight to Eradicate Smallpox*. Berkeley: University of California Press.

Foege, William H. 2018. *The Task Force for Child Survival: Secrets of Successful Coalitions*. Baltimore, MD: Johns Hopkins University Press.

Greene, Jeremy, Marguerite Thorp Basilico, Heidi Kim, and Paul Farmer. 2013. "Colonial Medicine and Its Legacies." In *Reimagining Global Health: An Introduction*, edited by Paul Farmer, Jim Yong Kim, Arthur Kleinman, and Matthew Basilico, 33–73. Los Angeles: University of California Press.

Harvey, Charles, Jillian Gordon, and Mairi Maclean. 2021. "The Ethics of Entrepreneurial Philanthropy." *Journal of Business Ethics* 171 (1): 33–49.

Hussein, Ghaiath, and Ross E.G. Upshur. 2013. "Ethical Challenges in Global Health Research." In *An Introduction to Global Health Ethics*, edited by Andrew D. Pinto and Ross E. G. Upshur, 103–116. New York: Routledge.

Kim, Jim Yong, Joyce V. Millen, Alec Irwin, and John Gershman, eds. 2000. *Dying For Growth: Global Inequality and the Health of the Poor*. Monroe, ME: Common Courage Press.

Lakoff, Andrew. 2010. "Two Regimes of Global Health." *Humanity: An International Journal of Human Rights, Humanitarianism, and Development* 1: 59–79.

Lane, Richard. 2012. "Bill Foege: Gentle Giant of Global Health." *Lancet* 379 (9835): 2419.

McGoey, Linsey. 2015. *No Such Thing as a Free Gift: The Gates Foundation and the Price of Philanthropy*. New York: Verso.

Mervis, Jeffrey. 2018. "U.S. Lawmakers Want NIH and CDC Foundations to Say More About Donors." *Science Insider*, June 29, 2018. Accessed 5/30/2023. https://www.science.org/content/article/us-lawmakers-want-nih-and-cdc-foundations-say-more-about-donors.

Packard, Randall M. 2016. *A History of Global Health: Interventions into the Lives of Other Peoples*. Baltimore, MD: Johns Hopkins University Press.

Pfeiffer, James, and Rachel Chapman. 2010. "Anthropological Perspectives on Structural Adjustment and Public Health." *Annual Review of Anthropology* 39: 149–165.

Rabinovitz, Jonathan. 1992. "CARE Headquarters to Move to Atlanta from Manhattan." *The New York Times*, September 20, 1992, 49, 1. https://www.nytimes.com/1992/09/20/nyregion/care-headquarters-to-move-to-atlanta-from-manhattan.html.

Reverby, Susan. 2009. *Examining Tuskegee: The Infamous Syphilis Study and Its Legacy*. Chapel Hill: University of North Carolina Press.

Rodney, Walter. 1972. *How Europe Underdeveloped Africa*. Washington, DC: Howard University Press.

Rosenberg, Mark L., Elisabeth S. Hayes, Margaret H. McIntyre, and Nancy Neill. 2010. *Real Collaboration: What It Takes for Global Health to Succeed*. Los Angeles: University of California Press.

Terris, Milton. 1999. "The Neoliberal Triad of Anti-Health Reforms: Government Budget Cutting, Deregulation, and Privatization." *Journal of Public Health Policy* 20 (2): 149–167.

Washington, Harriet A. 2006. *Medical Apartheid: The Dark History of Medical Experimentation on Black Americans from Colonial Times to the Present*. New York: Harlem Moon.

3 The Multimodal Poetics of Ethical Values

There's something better than science, and that's science with a moral compass
(Bill Foege[1])

In the 1980s, the introduction of neoliberal governance to public and global health led to the proliferation of secular non-profit organizations (NPOs), the increased reliance on public-private partnerships (PPPs), and the selective primary healthcare movement touted by Bill Foege and other global health experts. This resulted in a configuration of ethical values that has become central to global health. Like much of both "international health" of the mid-20th century and Christian missionary medicine, global health's ethical values are rooted in the idea of providing care to all, regardless of one's ability to pay for it (Brown 2014). Twenty-first-century iterations of these values have tended to avoid Christian proselytization, though the values are still based in Judeo-Christian conceptualizations of the self and of virtue (Black 2015). Anthropologist Didier Fassin (2012) argues that this sort of humanitarian reason—including concepts such as compassion and suffering—can motivate action in productive ways, but may also draw attention away from the violence, racism, and colonialism that marginalize communities and produce the conditions of suffering for which compassion is then a relevant response. In this chapter, I draw on this insight, balancing an analysis of the productive capacity of the ethical values of global health with a critique of the ways that these ethical values can reinscribe deeply problematic, colonially-rooted perspectives on aid and aid recipients.

For this project, I first discussed the topic of ethics, global health, and the global North with Dr. David G. Addiss. Dr. Addiss is a global health academic and practitioner with many years of experience working at CDC, the Task Force for Global Health, and Emory University. He has also published on the topic of ethics, and describes contemporary global health "as a manifestation of compassion" (Addiss 2016: 111). He generously agreed

DOI: 10.4324/9781003561019-3

to meet with me, consented to an interview, and decided that I should use his real name in published work.

In an email exchange before our initial meeting in May 2016, we agree to chat at what was the office of the Task Force for Global Health in downtown Decatur, Georgia (the organization later moved around the corner to a larger new office). It is a beautiful late spring day, not too hot, so I walk to the building from my house. It is subtle, an unassuming four- or five-story brick cube on the edge of the quaint downtown area of Decatur. So subtle, in fact, that I have lived for years in the city without realizing that it is home to one of the most significant global health NPOs in the country. Walking into the building, I am greeted by a friendly security guard. After I sign my name on a log sheet, he calls up Dr. Addiss on the phone and I sit down in a chair to wait in the small lobby of the building, picking up and flipping through the Task Force's glossy magazine-style annual report. The report includes a high-definition photograph of smiling African children on the cover. Soon Dr. Addiss comes to get me, and we walk up the stairs, past a small break room to his office.

One thing that interests me is how Dr. Addiss ended up at the Task Force. He tells me that the catalyst for him leaving CDC was what happened after September 11, 2001, when the attacks and their aftermath led to a shift in government priorities. Before that, he says, CDC felt like it was a bunch of former hippies roaming the halls in relaxed semi-professional clothing—essentially academics working on public and global health. After September 11, however, more of the organization's resources started being diverted to bioterrorism and the commissioned officer corps were expected to come to work more often in full military uniform. Addiss says that while he always knew he was technically working for a branch of the military, this became much more clearly a part of expectations for the work done at CDC after September 11. Nonetheless, he still collaborates closely with those at CDC, and many of those at the Task Force and other NPOs around town once worked with him at CDC, so there is a cohort of people that he sees regularly.

One interesting insight of Dr. Addiss' shares with me is that a surprisingly large number of the global health professionals whom he knows are the children of missionaries or church leaders (as he himself is). This could be framed as surprising in a context where, as he writes in his academic work, "[global health] remains wary of religion and its potential for divisiveness. The field is largely secular, pluralistic, science-based, results oriented, structurally complex, and predominantly funded by the public sector" (Addiss 2018: 339). In his own analysis of how ethics and religion may inform global health professionals' motivations, Addiss emphasizes spirituality and compassion. He separates an ethics of global health from the confines of Christianity and so potentially makes the field potentially more inclusive.

Still, it is important to note that the ethical tradition of global health can be traced historically to the work of Christian missionaries. In some ways, these Christian missionary medical roots were complementary to colonial medicine (Greene et al. 2013). Though many in global health hope they have moved beyond the worst parts of that tradition, current efforts to decolonize the field assert that certain aspects of colonial practices and ideologies persist in contemporary work. Anthropological scholarship concurs, discussing how the deployment of the concept of "global" in global health tends to privilege health professionals from high-income countries (Brada 2011, 2017). This and other implicit remnants of white supremacy may seep into health interventions:

> supremacy persists in the ways of seeing and assumptions that underpin global health practice. It is a supremacist way of seeing and doing when we entertain implicit hierarchical assumptions—for example, about the headquarters of a global health organisation being more important than its regional or country offices... And supremacy is enacted when a greater value is placed on research by [high-income countries] or distant experts than the knowledge of those with lived experience.
>
> (Abimbola and Pai 2020: 1627)

Here, if one substitutes the idea of "cultural standpoint" for "ways of seeing and assumptions that underpin" (see Duranti 2009b), Abimbola and Pai's editorial is primed for anthropological analysis of the cultural and discursive patterning of the field. In other words, their critique can be interpreted as being aimed at the *culture* of global health—a culture that cannot be fully separated from the scientific practices of the field (see also Jumab 2020). This culture was on full display in my first encounter at the Task Force—not as a direct result of the actions of Dr. Addiss or of the Task Force, but rather due to the social and historical setting in which those actions were produced and in which they make sense. The unassuming, neatly furnished and decorated office building in a high-income setting and the expensive annual report filled with numbers and figures but also with stories of aid and images of People of Color constitute the cultural realm in which key decisions get made. Yet, as mentioned in the introduction of this book, calls to decolonize the field may complicate such celebrations of the triumphs of the field's key concepts of partnership and collaboration.

In this chapter, I examine this tension, recognizing the deep interconnection between epistemic and ethical values in global health, as attested by Bill Foege's quote at the beginning of this chapter. I analyze how partnership and collaboration are deployed as ethical values within a pragmatic approach where the exigencies of actually providing care tend to outweigh philosophical or theoretical debates about issues such as the monetization of health or the role of private companies in global health. I discuss the construction of ethical values in global health stories across a range of public-facing examples: in promotional videos, global health websites, and recorded and observed discussion during global health symposia. Though it might seem that the ethical value at the root of collaboration is inclusion, a close look at how the term is employed and explained suggests that the underlying ethical value is, in reality, effectiveness. Here, in terms of Kockelman's (2020) theory of value, effectiveness in collaboration establishes relations between global health organizations in terms of relations between care provision and care recipients.

After a discussion of how global health professionals emplot collaboration and partnership, I then analyze the role of the multimodal poetics of racialized affect in these storytelling practices—in other words, how configurations of multimodal semiotic resources (e.g., music, images) implicitly and explicitly contribute to processes of racialization and marginalization that are associated with white supremacy (on racialized affect, see Berg and Ramos-Zayas 2015: 655; more on this below). In the context of global health storytelling, racialized affect may result in what I term racialized indexes of care.

The conclusions I reach in this chapter match those of a recent study of images that appeared in infectious disease gray literature published by global health organizations with headquarters in high-income countries (Charani et al. 2023). That study found that "the narrative currently depicted in imagery is one of power imbalances, depicting women and children from low-income and middle-income countries (LMICs) with less dignity, respect, and power than those from high-income countries" (Charani et al.: e155). In conjunction with the epistemic values associated with techno-optimism (discussed in Chapter 5), global health stories craft an imagined future in which donors and global health professionals have contributed to something good—namely, the betterment of humanity through the provision of health care—whereas those who cannot pay for that care themselves tend to be relegated to passive roles, positioned as aid recipients and sufferers rather than active participants in their own care or in the field of global health. Here I argue that though racialized affect may inspire philanthropists to donate to health causes, its continued use in global health storytelling hampers efforts to address inequities in the field.

Key Concepts: Ethical Values and Multimodal Poetics

Anthropological research on ethics examines how culture shapes the ways people think, feel, and talk about what one could, should, must, or might do. Ethical values, more specifically, are core principles or ideas that shape actions and their evaluation. These are part of cultural conceptions of what is good or desirable (Robbins 2012). As this description suggests, many anthropologists approach the study of ethics from a standpoint that is culturally—and to varying degrees morally—relativistic (Zigon 2008). In other words, scholars are not searching for the one true or best ethics, but rather are working to understand each community's distinct ethical values on their own terms.

Ethical values may range from verbally articulated discussions about ethics to unspoken habits that shape everyday life (Fader 2006; Garcia 2014; Zigon and Throop 2014). Some scholars label the former (reflection) as ethics, and the latter (habit) as morality. However, ethnographic research challenges this dichotomy, especially ethnographies of communication and everyday encounters (Lambek 2015: 5, fn 8). In particular, language provides numerous possibilities for the constitution of ethical values and reflexive discussion about them (Rumsey 2010; Sidnell 2010; Duranti 2009a). Indeed, the temporal unfolding of everyday discourse may involve intermediate, not-fully-coherent moments of reflection that fall somewhere in between reflection and habit. This suggests a continuum between the two (Throop 2003: 235). For ease of reference, in this book I use "ethics" to refer to the entire continuum.

In global health, ethical values are oriented toward the idea that those with resources *should* provide health care to those without resources. In the context of provision of care amid contemporary political and economic constraints, this is often operationalized as the values of effectiveness and collaboration. These ethical values establish relationships between global health NPOs from high-income countries and their "partners" from low- and middle-income countries in terms of relationships between healthcare actions and care recipient outcomes.

These ethical values are communicated in large part through multimodal poetics. The concept of a multimodal poetics links linguistic anthropological theorizations of multifunctionality and multimodality. Within a multifunctional analysis of language, the poetic function is one of multiple functions of language that are interrelated and co-constituted. In one classic model, for instance, the referential function is that aspect of language oriented toward the context of communication, while the phatic function is oriented toward contact among participants in an encounter. Poetics, however, is the aspect of language that is oriented toward aesthetics—toward the message for its own sake (Jakobson 1960). Poetics is significant in verbal art but is also as a part of all language use (Jakobson 1960: 356). The analysis of how people attend to the aesthetic contours of language during a story performance (Bauman 1975) should include not just the words that are spoken/signed, but also to a range of multimodal resources deployed, such as gesture, facial expression, body orientation, pitch contour, use of music, visual aids, the built environment, et cetera (Goodwin 1997; Haviland 2004; Goodwin 2018; Westmoreland 2022).[2] Mobilizing this understanding of language, in this chapter my analysis of multimodal poetics in global health storytelling reveals building blocks for the (re)creation of the field's ethical values.

Collaboration: The Ethics of Health for Most

Many global health professionals enact a "health for most" ethics—that is, a pragmatic ethics that points toward the notion that "health as a human right" while recognizing the reality of "health as a commodity" in much of the world today. Health as a human right (or health for all) involves providing health care to all persons regardless of their ability to pay for it. Health as a commodity means evaluating health care in terms of the market-value of that care, such that decisions about provision of care are made based on cost-effectiveness. In academic analyses of global health, these two stances are sometimes contrasted with one another and viewed as incompatible (Basilico et al. 2013). For instance, anthropologist-physician and global health luminary Paul Farmer (2015, 2003) was a famous advocate of health as a human right. He argued against applying the economic concept of "cost-effectiveness" to health care, insisting that governments and donors of high-income countries only deploy the rhetoric of cost-effectiveness when dealing with the world's poor and marginalized, and that wealthy nations have an ethical obligation to provide funding for care in low-income countries.

Not everyone agrees with Farmer's rejection of cost-effectiveness. For instance, Damian Walker (2019), a health economist working for the Bill and Melinda Gates Foundation and former associate professor at the Johns Hopkins School of Public Health, writes,

> Cost-effectiveness estimates and their component parts (costs, burden, coverage, efficacy and quality) are critical inputs to the [Gates] foundation's upstream and downstream decision-making and programmatic goals. In terms of strategy development, these data help inform areas we prioritize in terms of disease, interventions and research…[3]

While the Gates Foundation approach includes an evaluation of health interventions in economic terms (and terminology), it should be noted that there is still an underlying ethical motivation here, which is to care for the greatest number of people possible. The idea is that more lives will be saved if resources are allocated to care for as many people as possible (Paul Farmer had an answer to this too: that the rich have plenty of resources to provide care for all but spend those resources on other things).

In their everyday work, at least, global health professionals tend to eschew such debates and instead focus on how to accomplish each task at hand. This requires a certain flexibility. One must be able to work with a wide range of organizations that could have disparate goals and distinct orientations. The need for flexibility in working across organizations has been theorized by global health professionals as "collaboration." For instance, in the preface to a book on collaboration published by leaders of the Task Force for Global Health, Dr. William Foege explains,

> We have never been in a better position to extend a hand to people around the globe. With the resources of United Nations agencies; the foundations endowed by Rockefeller, Gates, Buffet, and Turner; Rotary International; pharmaceutical companies; bilaterals; multilaterals; and thousands of non-governmental organizations, we have an abundance to tap that is beyond anything we could have imagined fifty years ago. And the most important lesson of those fifty years is that collaboration is the best way to make those resources count.
>
> (Rosenberg et al. 2010: xi)

Foege's use of the "extend a hand" idiom (to offer support or assistance) invokes an ethics of providing care for those who cannot afford it. This idiom is rooted in Biblical passages about charity and love, while his conclusion about the "best way to make those resources count" points toward notions of cost-effectiveness. Collaboration is a theory about how to best manage the many organizations and sources of funding with an attention to cost-effectiveness as one important (but not the only important) goal (Rosenberg et al. 2010: 3).

The Values of Effectiveness and Collaboration

At the beginning of this project, in my efforts to access the global health community in Atlanta while "studying up" I soon realized that some of my students at Georgia State University—a school with many commuter students—had their own personal and familial connections to people working in the field (e.g., through parents, family friends). One such student was then-undergraduate Kristina Ellis. Ellis was one of five students with whom I was working on a qualitative coding and thematic analysis of global health websites. As part of our research efforts, some students, including Ellis, offered to interview global health professionals who they knew. Ellis decided to interview a family acquaintance who had worked in global health for many years.

Just Get on a Plane and Go

It is Fall 2018. Ellis is meeting with Dan Far, a former CDC epidemiologist, in his kitchen, with his wife Gail Far listening and contributing to the conversation. Recorder running, Ellis begins to ask Far questions about his work in public and global health. She mentions the different groups with which he worked and the initiatives in which he participated. After several minutes of discussion, Ellis prompts, "so, I mean, you named a lot of different organizations and agencies—"

Far replies, "right, and some of those organizations were also like the CDC Foundation."

"Right?" Ellis replies.

"CDC foundation is separate—outside of CDC." Far pauses dramatically. Then he abruptly shifts conversational gears, performing emphatic stress (indicated below with underlining) and sing-song voicing (which he uses to indicate tedious and/or ridiculous work). He does so as he imagines an epidemic scenario:

Dan Far: Ebola strikes… now… well, you think Dan Far is going to stay up all night and write a contract, get it pushed through, and sent out for bid, and get back three bids, and then have a conference, and figure out who gets the bid, and then have a protest against the bid, because somebody who lost the bid wants to win the bid, and so they put in an appeal… meanwhile, people are wanting to get on the airplane and go. CDC foundation gives them the money and they go. They're not hamstrung—

At this moment, Gail Far interjects, adding, "ready money."

Dan continues,

Dan Far: hamstrung by all that stuff.

Gail Far: Just write the check.

Dan Far: Write a check and do it. Get on the airplane and go. Don't even have to pick which friggin' airplane you go on. I'm serious. "Made in Amurrica" and you know what I mean, you know the rules, and the regulations? For doing contracts? And then you close me down? In September? Because of some political shenanigans, and Trump wants to build a wall? And now we're going to close down the CDC and all the government agencies with only essential personnel? And now the rest of us get sent home?

These last few sentences reference government shutdowns that have impacted CDC repeatedly over the past ten years due to political stalemates about the national budget. In fact, there were two partial government shutdowns in 2018, and in the news a third was being discussed as a distinct possibility at the time when this interview took place. Far's mention of "build a wall" refers to President Trump's threat to shut down the government if congress did not fund the building of a wall at the US/ Mexico border (an example of what Far refers to as political shenanigans).

This is just one of a number of examples that Far mentions as evidence of why it would be a mistake to rely on governmental agencies to quickly respond to a global health emergency. He also explains the complexity, slowness, and "the rules and the regulations" of the system of getting bids for government contracts, as well as the mandated preference for American companies and organizations. Far negatively evaluates these aspects of working within government institutions through his performative voicing of what might be described as a "rural conservative accent" stereotype when he says "made in Amurrica" [America]. In contrast, both Dan and Gail Far explain, with the CDC Foundation, you "just write the check... get on the plane and go."

This is a future-oriented story, an imaginative projection and prediction of what might happen. When another Ebola outbreak occurs, the story goes, the ability of global health professionals to effectively combat that outbreak would be hampered by the political and bureaucratic inefficiencies of a government agency. One possible response to such a problem might be to advocate for reforming CDC, but Far does not tell this sort of a story. Instead, he focuses on how to get things done now. Underlying this story is an ethics that asks: given the situation as it currently exists, what is the best way to provide care to the greatest number of people possible? It is this question that is at the root of the ethical value of effectiveness in global health.

Collaboration between CDC and the CDC Foundation is an example of what global health professionals and others describe as public-private partnerships (PPPs). Like Dan Far, many people that I talked to tended to valorize PPPs. This contrasts with some anthropological perspectives on neoliberalism and the subsequent effects of transnational NPOs on governmentality and sovereignty in low-income countries (as discussed in Chapter 2; Ferguson 1990, 2006; Fisher 1997). Writing about PPPs, Betsey Brada (2011) explains, "Neither exactly nongovernmental organizations (NGOs) nor bilateral aid, many partnerships claim to support existing state institutions in addition to improving health outcomes and 'building local capacity,' even as they seem to undermine these same institutions" (288–289). While this may be true, my experience with global health professionals such as Dan Far indicates that this statement should be put into the context of global health pragmatism and the pervasiveness of neoliberalism in the global economy. To many global health professionals, PPPs are often part of pragmatic attempts to provide care *despite* the defunding and weakening of governmental public health institutions.

Here there is tension between critiquing institutions as they now stand and not losing sight of the fact that there are lives at stake. As João Biehl (2016) states: "Analytical distance too easily becomes a sanctioned form of moral detachment that dooms people differently than humanitarian reason—but dooms them nonetheless" (134). Global health professionals with whom I spoke tended to adopt a humanitarian stance and to emphasize the practical concerns related to providing care to people. They argued that this is not an either/or situation. Countries need strong health systems and also sometimes need the flexibility provided by NPOs and private companies. This stance is rooted in an ethics of pragmatism linked to the value of effectiveness.

Getting Things Done on the Ground

While this discussion of PPPs paints a somewhat rosy picture of contemporary global health, other sources of discursive data raise some difficult questions about the pervasiveness of racialized inequities in representation in the field—inequities that are evident despite global health professionals' efforts to address these inequities. There is a wealth of available online data for the study of collaboration in global health. On YouTube, many global health NPOs maintain channels with dozens or even hundreds of videos on them. After watching dozens of these videos and speaking with global health communications experts, I realized that most of these videos can be divided into two core genres with regularly occurring conventions: (1) a lecture/symposium genre and (2) a promotional video (promo) genre. The lecture/symposium genre involves light editing and is usually a recording of a live global health event (discussed later in this chapter). The promo genre usually includes heavy editing, a soundtrack, and on-screen textual elements. These videos provide information about an organization or intervention's presentation of itself.

In 2017, the Task Force for Global Health posted a promo video about the concept of collaboration. As mentioned, "collaboration" was a key concept being promoted by the Task Force at that time. This video begins with a title slide and some introductory music that feels inspirational and non-intrusive, with what are called "sus chords" (discussed in detail below). After that, the video shifts to a head shot of Dr. Thorpe, a white woman[4] who was the Chair of the Board of Directors for the Task Force at the time that the video was created.[5] After a brief visual of Thorpe talking, the video shifts to a series of clips from Task Force activities while Thorpe continues speaking in a voice-over. Here is what Thorpe says:

Excerpt 6: The Task Force Model of Collaboration

Dr Thorpe: Collaboration is the cornerstone of the Task Force model and there is no public health problem in the world that can be solved without collaboration now. It's too complicated, there are too many interests that you cannot understand and know unless you've got a collaborative partner, you know—on the ground, working in the society where the problem is. There are organizations that have basically endorsed the Task Force model. Um, groups

> that are in the business of assessing who can get things done most effectively. The Gates Foundation is obviously one of those. They are—they are very careful about who they bring to the table to solve difficult problems; so are the big businesses, ah the big pharmaceutical houses. They don't turn over billions of dollars' worth of drug to solve a problem unless they—they have found a partner who can do the job. And I am so proud that the Task Force has been that place.

Dr. Thorpe focuses on the idea of solving problems. She emphasizes that all contemporary public health problems require collaboration (lines 01-03), that organizations such as the Gates Foundation are careful about who they work with to solve difficult problems (lines 08–09), and that pharmaceutical companies donate "billions of dollars' worth of drug to solve a problem" (lines 10–11)—with certain stipulations. These stipulations and this discussion about who to work with are connected, according to Thorpe, to getting things done effectively (line 07), and to being able to do the job (line 12). As with Dan Far's story about what happens when "Ebola strikes now," Thorpe's story revolves around an ethics of pragmatism. The stated reason to work with partners is because collaboration is necessary and because it works. And when global health works, more people receive the care that they need.

Dr. Thorpe describes some organizations as partners and collaborators. She states that one must have a collaborative partner "on the ground, working in the society where the problem is" (lines 04–05). Later, she mentions that pharmaceutical companies will not donate "billions of dollars' worth of drug" "unless they have found a partner" (lines 11–12). At that point, she names the Task Force as that partner (lines 12–13). The only named groups in this excerpt are the Task Force for Global Health, the Gates Foundation, and pharmaceutical companies. This deployment of the terms partnership and collaboration lays the groundwork for a story about the Task Force as an organization that works with the big players in global health (the Gates Foundation, the big pharmaceutical companies), and works effectively to solve health problems (as Thorpe states in line 07). In this example, the ethical value of effectiveness is linked to techno-optimism and to economic values: a pharmaceutical drug is presented as the solution to a hypothetical/future (health) problem; and the involvement of pharmaceutical companies is articulated in terms of "billions of dollars' worth of drug" (line 11).

Liable and Empowering Affect in "Collaboration"

This is not to say that the Task Force does not also work with organizations in the low-income countries where they coordinate intervention efforts, only that Dr. Thorpe does not mention those organizations while promoting the organization's ability to collaborate. However, the imagery and sound that accompany Dr. Thorpe's speech tell a different story. The visuals of this video match what I have seen in other videos and printed promotional materials of the Task Force from that time period (including the annual report mentioned at the beginning of this chapter). These visuals represent Task Force activities—and activities in global health interventions more generally—fairly well. The global health professionals who appear on screen and in frame are fairly diverse, including men and women, persons of color (POCs) and white persons.[6] Those seen to be receiving care, however, are all POCs. While potentially accurate in representing global health interventions, this division nonetheless reinforces and reinscribes the racialization of the field.

I do not mean for my analysis in this section to take away from the Task Force's excellent work to provide care or their efforts to present a public face of the organization that is diverse, nor do I mean to single this organization out. Rather, I hope to indicate the work that is still to be done to decolonize the stories that global health professionals tell. Indeed, decolonization of global health stories requires an analysis of the less explicit, less verbalized aspects of the stories (in other words, analysis of the multimodal poetics of these stories).

Ulla D. Berg and Ana Y. Ramos-Zayas (2015) theorize the concept of racialized affect, focusing on liable and empowering affect. About these ideas, the authors write,

> This conceptualization of "racialized affect," we propose, has two cornerstones. The first is "liable affect," that is, the affective practices that serve to racialize, contain, and sustain conditions of vulnerability and a constitutive element of subject formation for poor, migrant, and socially marginalized populations (and structured by the whiteness project extant in the contemporary United States). The second cornerstone is "empowering affect," that is, the affect associated with privilege and always-already perceived as complex, nuanced, and beyond essentialism. (662)

Both liable and empowering affect are on full display in the multimodal poetics of global health videos such as Dr. Thorpe's story about collaboration. Liable affect simplifies and essentializes. Images of People of Color—near shacks, dirt roads, and industrial sites (as in the visuals described below)—who are receiving medical care out in the open air have become iconic representations of poverty and suffering in the popular media of the United States and other high-income countries (Kleinman and Kleinman 1997). These images invoke not only an ethics of "health for all" but also a paternalistic orientation to charity rooted in the "white-savior industrial complex" (Cole 2012). Meanwhile, empowering affect is reproduced through narratives about effectiveness, efficiency, and partnership. It is not that liable affect is bad while empowering affect is good. Rather, the two work together to comprise racialized affect—which as a whole is problematic because it reproduces race-based inequities.

In global health discourses, liable and empowering affect play significant roles in the reproduction of what I term *racialized indexes of care*. In general terms, to index is to point toward something. The indexical is the aspect of language that is inexorably linked to context—that is, it is context dependent and context creating (Hanks 2001; Silverstein 2003; Nakassis 2018). In global health videos and images, Blackness is linked to care in ways that both rely on existing context and (re)create it: target populations of health interventions do tend to be People of Color (context dependence) and, by convention, in the discursive context of global health, images of People of Color who are not recognizably doctors or other health professionals create a sense of caring for those who cannot afford care themselves (context creation). It is in this sense that such images are racialized indexes of care.

In excerpt 6, after the title screen (featuring the Task Force logo) and a video clip of the Task Force headquarters in Decatur, this promo features a close-up of Dr. Thorpe speaking for about 15 seconds. Behind her, the background is blurry, but it is clear that she is speaking in some sort of an office. When she says, "collaborative partner" (line 04 in the excerpt), though, a series of videos flash on screen in succession. These appear to showcase a Task Force-led health intervention, perhaps somewhere in Africa. Neither the location nor the intervention are noted. There is a group of Black people sitting on wooden benches in a shaded dirt courtyard, waiting for what seems to be a consultation with POC service providers who are sitting at a wooden table. A White man in a wide-brimmed fedora and a man in a polo shirt and baseball cap look on. They might be Task Force employees.

Next the video shifts to a clip of a Black boy herding cattle (an archetypical image of Africa for American audiences), then to three women of color in what appears to be a Task Force office leaning over and pointing at a world map with outbreak hot spots indicated alongside text and numbers. A clip of the hallway sign of the Public Health Informatics Institute (in the Task Force headquarters) is followed by an image of a Black man and white woman in professional clothing walking down that hallway. Then the visual shifts to a white man in professional attire (Dr. Dave Ross, the former CEO of the Task Force) talking and pointing at an infographic on a TV screen. This is followed by a return to a close-up of Dr. Thorpe speaking until the end of the video, ending with the Task Force logo.

Dr. Thorpe's story is about the ways that the Task Force is able to be effective, to get things done in collaboration with the Gates Foundation and pharmaceutical companies (empowering affect). But at the same time, this hypercompetence is indexed through unlabeled clips of Black people—most likely in Africa (liable affect). These visuals reinforce the patterning of space between "here" and "there" (Brada 2011), a pattern that recurs across scales (Irvine and Gal 2000; Carr and Lempert 2016). As other scholars have noted, "storytelling participants engage in complex practices of scale-making within… tellings themselves" (Koven, Kramer, and Perrino 2024: 3). At the broadest level, "here" points to organizational headquarters in a high-income country while "there" points to the nation or region that is a target of a health intervention (in excerpt 6, Task Force headquarters in Decatur versus various locations in what appears to be East or West Africa). Scaling down, "here" is a country or regional office while "there" is the target community of an intervention (the target communities represented by various visuals of POC going about their lives or receiving care at a table outside). Empowering affect is linked to the ability of global health professionals, especially those from high-income countries, to move across these scales (e.g., the Task Force employees seen working "there" in African settings; the videos), while liable affect is linked to a lack of mobility on the part of aid recipients, and to a certain extent health professionals from low- and middle-income countries.

The Role of Racialized Indexes of Care in Techno-Optimism

This and other examples of racialized indexes of care persist despite the field's efforts toward equity. Perhaps one reason they do is because they are central to the construction of techno-optimistic stories. Another promo video, this one from an intervention called CHAMPS Health, provides a second example. CHAMPS (Child Health and Mortality Prevention Surveillance) is an Atlanta-based global health intervention funded by the Bill and Melinda Gates Foundation. The NPO collaborates with CDC, Emory University, and the Task Force for Global Health, among others. The stated motivation for CHAMPS is that there is not enough data on the causes of child mortality in low-income countries. The program responds to this lacuna at multiple sites around the globe, where doctors ask parents if they can take tissue samples from recently deceased children. Scientists then analyze those samples in conjunction with clinical data to try and ascertain each deceased child's cause of death. Taken in the aggregate, a key goal of CHAMPS is to use this data to craft more effective health interventions for children and infants in the future.

Like the Task Force for Global Health, CHAMPS has a robust website and YouTube channel. That channel includes a promo video for the organization. The promo video features an interview with an African health official, Dr. Samba Sow (Mali's Minister of Health and Public Hygiene).[7] The inclusion of Dr. Sow in this video—a step in the right direction—showcases the role of professionals from low- and middle-income countries in global health efforts and points toward both collaboration in general and PPPs more specifically.

The CHAMPS promo video features a narrator and musical accompaniment that plays over unlabeled silent videos, followed by clips of the interview with Dr. Sow with musical accompaniment). Here is what the narrator and Dr. Sow say at the conclusion of this video:

Excerpt 7: CHAMPS Health Promo (beginning at 4 min 21 sec of the video)

01 **Narrator:** This is the beginning of an effort that addresses a critical
02 knowledge gap. In the years ahead, addressing that gap should help prevent
03 childhood deaths and illness in places where far too many children die before
04 their fifth birthday.
05 **Dr. Samba Sow:** CHAMPS will help us make sure that our babies will
06 celebrate their fifth-year anniversary.

As in the Task Force video about collaboration (excerpt 7) and in many other global health promo videos, the music in excerpt 7 includes a basic, repetitive melodic line (ostinato) and a harmonic progression involving a suspended chord in a major key. In European classical and American popular music, major keys are usually interpreted as positive or happy, while suspended chords convey a sense of unresolved forward-facing movement. Jazz and popular music theorist Anton Schwartz (2013) describes such chords as feeling similar to navigating a ship on the open ocean:

> the nautical metaphor seems perfect: when you're out on the ocean, you may know that you are moving forward, and still you may have no sense of forward progress at all, judging by your proximity to the landmarks you see.

In conjunction with the video clips and linguistic content of this promo, the music might be interpreted as indicating a projection toward an as-yet-unfulfilled but hopeful future (in other words, optimism). Together, the musical and linguistic content relies on empowering affect and points toward ethical values of collaboration and effectiveness, indicating that the CHAMPS team will be able to overcome a complex worldwide problem.

Many of the visuals of this promo video, however, rely on liable affect. Before the clip of Dr. Samba Sow speaking, a number of unlabeled videos accompany a voice-over that describes the CHAMPS program. Those videos include Indian children smiling and pumping their fists as they sit or stand on top of a train that is quickly moving past shacks, dirt roads, and a concrete overpass; happy African children jumping up and down on a mostly dirt soccer field; and an African mother dressed with a traditional Maasai beaded headband, belt, and jewelry, who is smiling and holding a baby while two African women who are nurses smile and examine the child. Other than the nurses, there are only implicit connections between the video images and CHAMPS—or indeed, any health intervention. The people in the videos are children and they seem to be from low-income countries where CHAMPS is operating. These video clips may not need any explanation for some audiences because they have become iconic representations of poverty, suffering, and the promise of techno-optimistic interventions.

Significantly, the CHAMPS Health intervention involves discovering precisely what kills children and then, ostensibly, combatting those particular pathogens. Such an approach circumvents the need for structural change. An alternative approach might attempt to change the living conditions that currently cause child illness and death to be more prevalent in impoverished communities in low-income countries (or to simply increase the income of low-income parents). The Bill and Melinda Gates Foundation may have the best of intentions. Still, Bill Gates' fortune was made possible by globalized capitalist inequities that yielded low-cost production of electronics equipment—including the extremely low wage-work of West African miners who provided semi-precious metals for personal computers' central processing units (see Ferguson 2006: 36–37). It is not too much of a leap to say that the Gates Foundation is attempting to solve problems that its founder actually played a role in creating. And it is no surprise that the perspectives of philanthropists and corporate donors such as Bill and Melinda Gates would best match targeted interventions to fill gaps in care caused by the neoliberal economic policy that they actively support and benefit from, rather than advocacy for large-scale structural changes that would threaten the business models by which they attained their own success.

The reliance on liable and empowering affect in global health promo videos such as these also demonstrates the role of storytelling in the imaginative constitution of social worlds. Imagined futures are constrained by existing genres, communicative conventions, and socioeconomic patterns. To circulate, stories about existing and potential health interventions need to not only make sense but also be compelling to target audiences, which include global health professionals, philanthropists, and corporate donors. In order for global health NPOs to be effective—to enact an ethics of pragmatism—they need to attract interest, direct people's efforts, and obtain funding. And targeted techno-optimistic interventions that provide care for impoverished Black people, Indigenous people, and People of Color (BIPOC) living in low-income countries are appealing to donors.

Affective Effectiveness in Symposia

These and other promotional videos posted on YouTube link effectiveness—as an ethical value associated with the terms collaboration and partnership—with techno-optimism. Such linkages are also made in other genres of global health discourses, particularly in global health symposia. Symposia are an important data source because the primary audiences for these events and recordings are other global health professionals and students. In the Atlanta metropolitan area prior to the start of the COVID-19 pandemic, global health symposia that were open to the public were fairly frequent (occurring a few times per year). I attended and took fieldnotes at three of these events. Many symposia were also professionally video-recorded and uploaded to YouTube. I thus was able to also watch and analyze several other events online. After promotional videos, symposia videos were the most common genre of video that I found on the YouTube channels of global health organizations.

"Africans Are Used to Getting Tested"

One of the events that I was able to attend in person was titled "Mobile to Multiplex: Accelerating Innovation in Global Diagnostics." This symposium was co-hosted by the Task Force for Global Health and the Georgia Global Health Alliance. The event was held at the Task Force's headquarters. While it was recorded and was meant to be posted online, unfortunately a technical issue resulted in the recording being damaged. Here, I rely on my fieldnotes and experiences at the event. What follows is a brief description.

It is April 2019. Upon arrival at the front of the Task Force's brand-new headquarters, I walk into a glassed-in vestibule. There is a ringer to buzz the front desk, but many people are going in, so the door is open. I walk past a large circular desk that sits in the middle of a reception area. Everything looks shiny and fancy. Moving to a welcome table, I speak with an intern, who picks my nametag out from about 75 or so and hands it to me. I also grab a brochure of the Task Force's 2018 yearly report and a flier for today's event. The intern directs me further back into the building, where a snack buffet has been set up next to a large conference room with three screens, projectors, and seating areas.

I browse the buffet tables. While waiting for the event to start, I hear terms and phrases such as "collaboration," "our foundation's in Belgium," and "did you get the money?!" (this last one was shouted out). I also encounter one of my neighbors, who tells me that she now works for the Task Force. As I walk around, I glance at people's nametags to get a sense of their professional affiliations. It is a mishmash that represents most of the different kinds of organizations involved in global health, including the Task Force, other Atlanta-area non-profits, Emory University, CDC, a few businesses, and other colleges and universities such as Georgia State University, Morehouse College, and Georgia Tech. It is a fairly diverse crowd, though there are more men than women and more White people than People of Color.

I sit in a back corner of the large conference room where I can observe and take notes easily. The event's formal presentation begins. The presentation relies heavily on empowering affect, describing how a technological innovation is going to solve a complex problem in the provision of care to those who are unable to pay for that care. The keynote speaker, Dr. Daniel Fletcher (a white man who is a professor of bioengineering at UC Berkeley), tells a story about how he developed the "LoaScope." The LoaScope is a special phone case—a microscope, in effect—that attaches to a mobile phone. A slot in the phone case provides a space to put a medical slide with a droplet of blood. Bluetooth communication between the case and a phone app triggers tiny slide movements so that the phone-microscope can capture many short videos of different slide regions. Then the app uses algorithms to analyze those videos to look for the sorts of microscopic movement that indicate the presence of a particular kind of parasite called Loa loa (aka African eye worm). This diagnosis is important: a medicine used to treat other parasites common in West Africa can cause severe complications for those infected with Loa loa such that individuals diagnosed with Loa loa infection must not take the medicine. One of Fletcher's primary stated goals for the development of this mobile-phone app is to bypass the need for more expensive testing or cadres of trained medical professionals in areas of the world without robust or well-funded health systems. In other words, his techno-optimistic intervention would involve targeted intervention but not include an investment in structural change to expand or strengthen the health systems of West African nations.

After Fletcher's presentation, the symposium shifts gears to a panel discussion. The panel includes four white global health experts (two men and two women) associated with CHAMPS, the Georgia Institute of Technology, Emory University, and the Task Force for Global Health. The conversation ranges across a number of topics and involves audience participation. One question in particular from an audience member—who is a POC—gets my attention because it focuses on a potential ethical issue related to economic inequities and cultural difference. He asks, how it can be known whether potential patients will consent to have their blood drawn? One of the panelists quickly replies, "Africans are used to getting tested for malaria."

This answer shocks me—it is a dismissive hyper-generalization about a huge population living across a vast continent consisting of over fifty countries, not to mention the fact that malaria is not endemic to all of Africa (though it is endemic to the parts of West Africa where Loa loa is also most prevalent). The panelist's reply deploys liable affect, simplifying the lives of and disempowering Africans. While it is true that this statement goes unchallenged by the hundreds of global health professionals in the room, this cannot be taken as an indication of Dr. Fletcher's perspective or the perspective of others at the event—perhaps due to a general professional ethos of non-confrontation.

The (Mis)Uses of Accompaniment

A similar lack of confrontation occurred in an example taken from another symposium that was recorded and posted online. In the excerpt below, a speaker misuses an anti-racist concept—accompaniment—in a way that invokes racialized indexes of care. And he does so in front of the person who has done the most to develop the concept of accompaniment for global health. Anthropologist/physician/NPO leader Paul Farmer wrote extensively on accompaniment to advocate for a type of self-leveling that he felt should occur in public and global health contexts that included meeting each patient where they currently are (Farmer and Gutiérrez 2013). For instance, In his early HIV treatment efforts in Haiti, Farmer responded to patients' needs by providing financial and nutritional support, visiting patients in their homes, and helping with childcare and rent (Farmer 2013: 227).

Accompaniment, which is rooted in liberation theology, will be discussed in greater detail in Chapter 7. Here, it should be noted that accompaniment describes ethical engagement of health professionals from high-income countries with organizations, professionals, and patients from low-income countries. Additionally, it is persons from high-income countries who are meant to be doing the accompanying, "supporting developing country partners—public and private—until they have the capacity to deliver services and improve livelihoods in the long term" (Weigel, Basilico, and Farmer 2013: 294).

In September of 2015, the Task Force hosted an event to celebrate their thirty-year anniversary. Afterward, a recording of the symposium was posted on YouTube, titled "Panel Discussion: A Celebration of Three Decades of Contributions to Global Health."[8] While I did not attend this event in person, the recording of the event enables its analysis as an example of the in-person (aka "face-to-face") dynamics of global health storytelling.

The symposium included a roundtable discussion with Dr. Paul Farmer (co-founder of Partners in Health), Dr. Bill Foege, Dr. Jim Kim (World Bank President and co-founder of Partners in Health), Dr. Matshidiso [Tshidi] Moeti (World Health Organization Regional Director for Africa, formerly worked for the Botswana Ministry of Health, UNAIDS, and UNICEF), and moderator Dr. Mark Rosenberg (Task Force CEO at the time of the event and former CDC leader). Earlier, Rosenberg had gone through the list of participants, introducing each speaker at length with mention of their accomplishments (including Dr. Moeti). And just prior to excerpt 8, Rosenberg had described some of Moeti's accomplishments in more detail.

Continuing this description, Rosenberg tells a brief story about who Moeti is and what she has done:

Excerpt 8: Panel Discussion (starting at 18 min 41 sec)

01 Mark Rosenberg: she's from Botswana and she's served in administrative
02 positions for the ministry of health there, and in her new role she has
03 committed to work with transparency, something extraordinarily important in
04 Africa, efficiency and equity. And she's committed to bringing universal
05 healthcare coverage to Africa, and she brings hope and understanding to the
06 health issues that face the people of Africa in a new and very, very exciting
07 way. And Paul [Farmer] has talked about accompaniment, an extraordinary
08 idea, and Tshidi is here, I think it's no small chance, that she's accompanying
09 us in talking about this, she needs to be part of this, and we're delighted to
10 have you here, Tshidi, thank you.

It is clear from this and the larger discussion from which the excerpt is drawn that Rosenberg has great respect for Moeti and her work. He deploys core ethical values of global health in his description, including efficiency (line 04)—notably alongside equity—and the concept of health for all ("universal healthcare coverage," lines 04–05).

However, a problem arises for Rosenberg when he introduces the concept of accompaniment (lines 07–09), referencing Farmer's articulation of this idea. Rosenberg says, "she's accompanying us in talking about this." Notably, Farmer's version of this concept does not include one elite global health professional speaking to another elite global health professional—regardless of the individuals' origins. So why might Rosenberg use the concept in this way? Liable affect seems to seep into Rosenberg's story about Moeti's background and contributions to global health: rather than being rooted in an in-depth analysis of existing socioeconomic inequities in relationships between global health partners, accompaniment becomes simplified into something that is applicable when working with Africans and other People of Color. And yet Paul Farmer does not visibly react or respond—perhaps not wanting to derail the introduction.

Friends in High Places

This is not the only moment in the panel discussion where neither the audience nor the other panelists respond to Rosenberg's comments. About two and a half minutes earlier, Rosenberg had told a story about Jim Kim and Paul Farmer's early involvement in multi-drug-resistant tuberculosis (MDR-TB) treatment in Peru. He described how Kim and Farmer had spent almost 100,000 dollars in their efforts, and how no one wanted to fund their work because it was considered to be too expensive—not an effective use of limited funding (using the logic of cost-effectiveness).

Rosenberg's story continues. Kim calls Rosenberg and says that they need a grant for a million dollars to keep their program successful enough to "show the world that it works." Rosenberg sets up a meeting with Bill Foege, who is working at the Gates Foundation at that time. After a grant proposal and some back-and-forth, the Gates Foundation gives Kim and Farmer a grant for forty-four and a half million dollars.

Foege interrupts, asking, "Can I add a note?"

"Sure," Mark replies.

"Ah, this grant proposal went to Bill Gates. He sent it back to me and said, 'aren't they padding the budget?'"

Members of the audience laugh at this question.

Foege continues, "And so, ah, which they were, but…" Audience members laugh some more. Then Foege says,

> But I sent him a copy of the New Yorker Magazine that talked about "Paul had only one suit, and it was a black suit because he tended to get ink stains on it," and I said people with one suit don't usually pad the budget.

The audience laughs again.

Foege smiles and emphasizes, "And he approved it!" Audience members laugh some more. At this point, Rosenberg takes the lead as moderator again, still smiling, and explains, "friends in high places sometimes make all the difference." The audience does not laugh at Rosenberg's summary.

Jokes are some of the most difficult cultural content for anthropologists to explain because they rely heavily on implicitly shared knowledge and beliefs (Black 2012). Some familiarity with the culture of global health is necessary to understand why the audience laughs at Foege's comments but not Rosenberg's. It is true that in his joking performance, Foege's timing was impeccable, as he paused and waited at three moments for audience laughter. And his delivery was subtle—nearly deadpan but with a hint of a smile. In addition, much of the humor of his joke relied on a widely shared perception among global health professionals and medical anthropologists that Paul Farmer was a morally upright crusader for the health of the poor who had little concern for his own wealth or status. This perception has been reinforced by numerous journalistic accounts of his work, most notably Tracy Kidder's (2003) book, *Mountains beyond Mountains: The Quest of Dr. Paul Farmer, a Man Who Would Cure the World.*

As Foege spoke, audience members laughed first at the idea that a person like Paul Farmer would do something as ethically dubious as exaggerate the numbers in a budget. Next, they laughed at Foege's quip that of course they were padding the budget. Here, one implicit understanding is that if Farmer and Kim were actually doing so, it would be in order to better help the world's poor, not for their own gain. After this, the audience laughed at the statement that people with one suit don't usually pad the budget, in further recognition of Farmer's celebrated selfless nature. Finally, they laughed when they learned that the gambit worked, with Farmer and Kim securing the resources they needed with help from Foege.

In contrast, only silence followed Rosenberg's comment that friends in high places make a difference. One way to interpret this silence is that audience members did not recognize Rosenberg's comment as a joke and did not agree that Paul Farmer could be characterized as engaging in nepotistic wheeling and dealing. However, they had just laughed at the idea of Farmer padding a budget. Another interpretation—the one that I think is most likely correct—is that the audience was reacting to how the comment contradicted the idea that *effective* interventions will receive financial support because they *deserve* support. Rosenberg's statement suggested that the ability to be effective in providing care (Rosenberg had said that Kim and Farmer needed a million dollars to be able to be successful, to show the world that their program worked) was dependent not on the inherent worth of the intervention but rather on the whims of a wealthy benefactor. Rosenberg was "saying the quiet part out loud," discussing something that the global health professionals in the audience may have objected to or not wanted to confront. This may be precisely because contemporary global health requires two potentially contradictory things to be laminated onto one another: first, that wealthy philanthropists and other donors like and want to support a given health intervention; and, second, that global health NPOs do what is most effective based on the science (data-driven interventions).

Conclusion

Liable and empowering affect in global health storytelling are not only harmful to efforts toward equity but also inaccurate. Too often the valuing of scientific expertise (to be discussed in Chapter 5) entails the elevation of doctors and epidemiologists as decision-makers and a discounting of the significant knowledge and experience of aid recipients—sometimes including the dismissal or minimization of the expertise of doctors and other health professionals from low- and middle-income countries. I saw this firsthand when I conducted ethnographic fieldwork in South Africa Patient-activists living with HIV had ideas for ways to improve health interventions but did not have the financial support to implement them. For instance, one group member hoped to start a food bank for her community. While this might be seen as outside the purview of an HIV intervention, she noted that many anti-retroviral medications (ARVs [for treating HIV]) were required to be taken with food. Thus, providing ARVs to people experiencing food insecurity was ineffective without also providing food. But this sort of idea would likely never make its way into a grant proposal written 8,000 miles away without her input.

Still, it is important to emphasize that global health ethics are pragmatic in nature and oriented toward providing care for as many people as possible who are unable to pay for that care themselves. Global health professionals evaluate how they should proceed in order to accomplish their goals given the way things are now amid the need to solicit funding for their work. Here, effectiveness is a core ethical value. It establishes relations between partners/collaborators in terms of relations between the provision of health care and the recipients of that care. These values are (re)constituted through stories in which the multimodal poetics of liable and empowering affect yield racialized indexes of care (indexes that may appeal to donors). In this way, despite the stated commitment of many global health professionals to equity and anti-racism, the constitution of these ethical values nonetheless (re)imagines a world that is inequitable.

Relying on grants and donations to do their work, global health professionals are in a difficult position. As a concept, effectiveness is linked not only to epistemic values to be discussed in Chapter 5 (most notably, expertise, efficacy of treatment, biomedicalization, and spatial generalization) but also to the economic values associated with the circulation of stories and fundraising (as will be discussed in the next chapter). Simply put, it is important for NPOs to craft stories that appeal to corporate and philanthropic donors, and, indirectly, to the public at large. Despite insistence that financial or social gain is not the motivation for giving, donors do gain from their activities in ways that are only possible when donors are able to reference or be linked to the compelling stories told by their chosen NPOs. A challenge to global health professionals, then, is to decolonize the stories that they tell about their work in such a way that their stories continue to appeal to donors. Successful examples of such storytelling do exist. Those stories will be discussed in Chapters 6 and 7. First, though, the book explores another type of values that is significant in global health: economic values.

Notes

1 https://www.youtube.com/watch?v=4Ax_ngXdZM4. Accessed 3/9/2023 (2 min 27 sec).

2 Recent scholarship has emphasized multimodal anthropology to describe the use of recordings, social media, and digital software to capture ethnographic data and represent culture in research products (Westmoreland 2022). While attending to the contributions of this new work and its connections to the history of visual anthropology, it is important to also recognize the strong tradition of multimodality that is decades old in linguistic anthropology, especially with regard to the analysis of communication and the presentation of results.

3 https://www.gatesfoundation.org/ideas/articles/health-economist-global-health-financing. Accessed 2/6/2023.

4 The race-based descriptors here are my own perceptions (I have no way of knowing how the people in the video identify). I include them here because potential audience perceptions of race in these videos are a significant aspect of the analysis.

5 https://www.youtube.com/watch?v=hBU42r4CNTo. Accessed 2/9/2023.

6 These race-based categories may not be relevant in all parts of the world where global health organizations work. However, I describe visuals of people in promotional videos using these categories because they do tend to be relevant for the intended primary audiences of the videos as discussed earlier.

7 https://www.youtube.com/watch?v=9S8k1Nsu6fc. Accessed 2/21/2023.

8 https://www.youtube.com/watch?v=24YkghgecNo&t=1027s. Accessed 2/28/2023.

References

Abimbola, Seye, and Madhukar Pai. 2020. "Will Global Health Survive its Decolonization?" *The Lancet* 396 (10263): 1627–1628.

Addiss, David G. 2016. "Globalisation of Compassion: The Example of Global Health." In *Why Love Matters: Values in Governance*, edited by Scherto Gill and David Cadman, 107–119. New York: Peter Lang.

Addiss, David. 2018. "Spiritual Themes and Challenges in Global Health." *Journal of Medical Humanities* 39 (3): 337–348.

Basilico, Matthew, Jonathan Weigel, Anjali Motgi, Jacob Bor, and Salmaan Keshavjee. 2013. "Health For All? Competing Theories and Geopolitics." In *Reimagining Global Health: An Introduction*, edited by Paul Farmer, Jim Yong Kim, Arthur Kleinman and Matthew Basilico, 74–110. Berkeley: University of California Press.

Bauman, Richard. 1975. "Verbal art as Performance." *American Anthropologist* 77 (2): 290–311.

Berg, Ulla D., and Ana Y. Ramos-Zayas. 2015. "Racializing Affect: A Theoretical Proposition." *Current Anthropology* 56 (5): 654–677.

Biehl, Joao. 2016. "Theorizing Global Health." *Medicine Anthropology Theory* 3 (2): 127–142.

Black, Steven P. 2012. "Laughing to Death: Joking as Support amid Stigma for Zulu-speaking South Africans Living with HIV." *Journal of Linguistic Anthropology* 22 (1): 87–108.

Black, Steven P. 2015. "The Morality of Performance: HIV Disclosure in Speech and Song in South Africa." *Ethos* 43 (3): 247–266.
Brada, Betsey Behr. 2011. "'Not Here': Making the Spaces and Subjects of 'Global Health' in Botswana." *Culture, Medicine, and Psychiatry* 35 (2): 285–312.
Brada, Betsey Behr. 2017. "Exemplary or Exceptional? The Production and Dismantling of Global Health in Botswana." In *Global Health and Geographical Imaginaries*, edited by Clare Herrick and David Reubi, 40–53. New York: Routledge.
Brown, Peter J. 2014. "Religion and Global Health." In *Religion as a Social Determinant of Global Health*, edited by Ellen Idler, 273–297. Oxford: Oxford University Press.
Carr, E. Summerson, and Michael Lempert, eds. 2016. *Scale: Discourse and Dimensions of Social Life*. Oakland: University of California Press.
Charani, Esmita, Sameed Shariq, Alexandra M. Cardoso Pinto, Raabia Farooqi, Winnie Nambatya, Oluchi Mbamalu, Seye Abimbola, and Marc Mendelson. 2023. "The Use of Imagery in Global Health: An Analysis of Infectious Disease Documents and a Framework to Guide Practice." *Lancet Global Health* 11 (1): E155–E164.
Cole, Teju. 2012. "The White-Savior Industrial Complex." *The Atlantic*, March 21, 2012.
Duranti, Alessandro. 2009a. "The Force of Language and its Temporal Unfolding." In *Language in Life and a Life in Language: Jacob Mey – A Festschrift*, edited by Kenneth Turner and Bruce Fraser, 63–71. Bingley: Emerald Group Publishers.
Duranti, Alessandro. 2009b. "The Relevance of Husserl's Theory to Language Socialization." *Journal of Linguistic Anthropology* 19 (2): 205–226.
Fader, Ayala. 2006. "Learning Faith: Language Socialization in a Community of Hasidic Jews." *Language in Society* 35 (2): 205–229.
Farmer, Paul. 2003. *Pathologies of Power: Health, Human Rights, and the New War on the Poor*. Los Angeles: University of California Press.
Farmer, Paul. 2013. *To Repair the World: Paul Farmer Speaks to the Next Generation*. Los Angeles: University of California Press.
Farmer, Paul. 2015. "Who Lives and Who Dies: Paul Farmer on the Inequities of Healthcare Funding." *London Review of Books* 37 (3): 17–20.
Farmer, Paul, and Gustavo Gutiérrez. 2013. *In the Company of the Poor: Conversations between Dr. Paul Farmer and Gustavo Gutiérrez*. Maryknoll, NY: Orbis Books.
Fassin, Didier. 2012. *Humanitarian Reason: A Moral History of the Present*. Translated by Rachel Gomme. Los Angeles: University of California Press.
Ferguson, James. 1990. *The Anti-Politics Machine: "Development," Depoliticization and Bureaucratic Power in Lesotho*. New York: Cambridge University Press.
Ferguson, James. 2006. *Global Shadows: Africa in the Neoliberal World Order*. Durham, NC: Duke University Press.
Fisher, William. 1997. "Doing Good? The Politics and Antipolitics of NGO Practices." *Annual Review of Anthropology* 26: 439–464.
Garcia, Angela. 2014. "The Promise: On the Morality of the Marginal and the Illicit." *Ethos* 42 (1): 51–64.

Goodwin, Marjorie. 1997. “By-play: Negotiating Evaluation in Story-telling.” In *Towards a Social Science of Language: Papers in honour of William Labov*, edited by Gregory R. Guy, John Baugh, Deborah Schiffrin, and Feagin Crawford, 77–102. Philadelphia, PA: John Benjamins.

Goodwin, Charles. 2018. *Co-Operative Action*. New York: Cambridge University Press.

Greene, Jeremy, Marguerite Thorp Basilico, Heidi Kim, and Paul Farmer. 2013. “Colonial Medicine and Its Legacies.” In *Reimagining Global Health: An Introduction*, edited by Paul Farmer, Jim Yong Kim, Arthur Kleinman, and Matthew Basilico, 33–73. Los Angeles: University of California Press.

Hanks, William F. 2001. “Indexicality.” In *Key Terms in Language and Culture*, edited by Alessandro Duranti, 119–121. Malden, MA: Blackwell.

Haviland, John. 2004. “Gesture.” In *A Companion to Linguistic Anthropology*, edited by Alessandro Duranti, 197–221. Malden, MA: Wiley-Blackwell.

Irvine, Judith, and Susan Gal. 2000. “Language Ideology and Linguistic Differentiation.” In *Regimes of Language: Ideologies, Polities, and Identities*, edited by Paul V. Kroskrity, 35–83. Santa Fe, NM: School of American Research.

Jakobson, Roman. 1960. “Concluding Statement: Linguistics and Poetics.” In *Style and Language*, edited by T. A. Sebeok, 350–377. Cambridge, MA: MIT Press.

Jumab, Desmond T. 2020. “How (not) to Write about Global Health.” *BMJ Global Health* 5: e003164. https:// doi.org/10.1136/bmjgh-2020-003164.

Kidder, Tracy. 2003. *Mountains Beyond Mountains: The Quest of Dr. Paul Farmer, a Man who Would Cure the World*. New York: Random House Trade Paperbacks.

Kleinman, Arthur, and Joan Kleinman. 1997. “Cultural Appropriations of Suffering in Our Own Times.” In *Social Suffering*, edited by Arthur Kleinman, Veena Das, and Margaret Lock, 1–23. Los Angeles: University of California Press.

Koven, Michele, Elise Kramer, and Sabina M. Perrino. 2024. “Introduction to ‘Scaling Stories: Narratives and the Dialogic Regimentation of Scales’.” *Discourse Studies* 1–9. https://journals.sagepub.com/doi/10.1177/14614456241276718

Lambek, Michael. 2015. “The Ethical Condition.” In *The Ethical Condition: Essays on Action, Person, and Value*, edited by Michael Lambek, 1–39. Chicago, IL: University of Chicago.

Nakassis, Constantine V. 2018. “Indexicality’s Ambivalent Ground.” *Signs and Society* 6 (1): 281–304.

Robbins, Joel. 2012. “Cultural Values.” In *A Companion to Moral Anthropology*, edited by Didier Fassin, 117–132. Malden, MA: Wiley-Blackwell.

Rosenberg, Mark L., Elisabeth S. Hayes, Margaret H. McIntyre, and Nancy Neill. 2010. *Real Collaboration: What It Takes for Global Health to Succeed*. Los Angeles: University of California Press.

Rumsey, Alan. 2010. “Ethics, Language, and Human Sociality.” In *Ordinary Ethics: Anthropology, Language, and Action*, edited by Michael Lambek, 105–122. New York: Fordham University Press.

Schwartz, Anton. 2013. *Understanding Sus Chords*. https://antonjazz.com/2013/03/sus-chords/ Accessed 2/2/2020.

Sidnell, Jack. 2010. "The Ordinary Ethics of Everyday Talk." In *Ordinary Ethics: Anthropology, Language, and Action*, edited by Michael Lambek, 123–139. New York: Fordham University Press.

Silverstein, Michael. 2003. "Indexical Order and the Dialectics of Sociolinguistic Life." *Language and Communication* 23 (3–4): 193–229.

Throop, C. Jason. 2003. "Articulating Experience." *Anthropological Theory* 3 (2): 219–241.

Walker, Damian. 2019. "Measuring the Value of Health." *Ideas*. https://www.gatesfoundation.org/ideas/articles/health-economist-global-health-financing.

Weigel, Jonathan, Matthew Basilico, and Paul Farmer. 2013. "Taking Stock of Foreign Aid." In *Reimagining Global Health: An Introduction*, edited by Paul Farmer, Arthur Kleinman, Jim Kim and Matthew Basilico, 287–301. Berkeley: University of California Press.

Westmoreland, Mark R. 2022. "Multimodality: Reshaping Anthropology." *Annual Review of Anthropology* 51: 173–194.

Zigon, Jarrett. 2008. *Morality: An Anthropological Perspective*. New York: Berg.

Zigon, Jarrett, and C. Jason Throop. 2014. "Moral Experience: Introduction." *Ethos* 42 (1): 1–15.

4 The Economic Value of Story Circulation

In February 2020, I meet Scott in a crowded popular coffee shop in one of the newly renovated (gentrified) parts of Atlanta. A white American man in his forties, Scott has worked in global health for over twenty years. In one of his online profiles, he describes himself as a partnership builder who could "engage and mobilize stakeholders." As someone who makes a living commodifying communication, he has well-developed theories, informed by his education and professional training, about how to best employ different aspects of global health discourses to meet his organization's goals. He is working from home today, and the coffee shop is closer than his office.

I am worried that the noisy din of chatty customers and espresso machines might limit my ability to record our interview on my cell phone, but I do a quick check and find that I can hear both of us speaking clearly. As we begin our conversation, Scott focuses on a website redesign he recently completed for the organization for which he works. He explains some of the flaws in his non-profit organization's (NPO's) communications program—he jokes that the communications program was non-existent before he got there—and he discusses some of the initial brainstorming that went into the website redesign. He is happy with the work he has done to improve it.

Then Scott says (3 min 39 sec),

> but even before we went down that road, we also looked at "what were our communications objectives?" So, what business goals of the [organization] could communications help support? So top of that list was fundraising, as it is for most any NGO.

Scott laughs at this statement. Though I laugh with him, I am not entirely sure what is funny about this—it just seems accurate to me. However, as discussed in the previous chapter, perhaps it is humorous and a bit uncomfortable to explicitly draw attention to the economics of philanthropy.

DOI: 10.4324/9781003561019-4

Later, Scott mentions that the narratives that his organization creates are "designed to address those interests of our audiences when they are considering us as a partner," noting the Gates Foundation as one of those potential partners. This confirms my tentative analysis of audiences and the creation of websites, YouTube videos, and other public-facing communication. NPOs need donations to survive, and their glossy pamphlets, YouTube channels, and elaborate websites are a key part of how they solicit donations.

But Scott complicates this understanding. He says, "when I think about communications it's, you know, broad communications like a website does but it's also one-on-one communications, and you need to have an effective story" (Interview 02-07-2020, 17 min 23 sec). He tells me that YouTube videos, websites, and symposia help create a streamlined story of his organization that is not just for funding. The NPO's story, repeated with alterations across platforms, also helps current employees develop a shared vision of the organization and helps to recruit future employees. Scott mentions instances when online videos have been played for potential donors and corporate "partners" in face-to-face meetings—not as a way to immediately secure funding but rather to generate general interest in his NPO. This is part of building partnerships and mobilizing stakeholders (as his professional profile states). The YouTube videos are part of his process of crafting stories about what his organization has done, but also about creating a vison of what his organization could optimistically do in the future if given the right resources with the right employees.

A few minutes earlier in our interview, Scott had ruminated on the non-linear nature of communications and its relationship to funding:

Excerpt 9: Institutional Narrative (starting at 11 min 27 sec)

> Scott: I always tell [the head of the NPO] that communications is not a linear cause and effect—because we have a nice website, the Gates Foundation is contacting us for this funding opportunity. It's part of a larger awareness building campaign that, you know, covers everything from digital assets to personal relationships. And that's the other piece of this; we want to arm our program directors and our staff with the information that <u>they</u> need in order to advocate to funders for new programs or to sustain the existing programming as well. So we are intentional about that—that our new institutional narrative is socialized with our staff, so that they can tell it to those high value audiences.

This is a clear articulation of why NPOs tell stories about their work, or at least why they do so according to a communications director. In his statement, the demonstrative pronoun "those" ("tell [the new institutional narrative] to **those** high value audiences") may refer to Scott's earlier mention of the Gates Foundation. The Gates Foundation is an example of the sort of audience to which a communications director wants his NPO's employees to tell carefully crafted stories. This is done in order to promote a relationship that might eventually lead to a donation.

This chapter is about the core principles that global health professionals such as Scott have deemed central to the goal of telling stories to such "high value audiences." The chapter is not about on the core economic values (e.g. "efficiency") that underpin global health (for a discussion of those values, see Basilico et al. 2013; Mei 2017). Instead, I write about how economic value (i.e., monetary income) is generated through storytelling, examining how global health NPOs attract donations through the circulation of stories. Global health professionals utilize specific communicative strategies to generate interest in their NPOs' efforts with the ultimate goal of attracting donors.

There are three core values that are linked to these strategies: transparency, successfulness, and narrative virtuosity. Here, transparency refers to the manner in which NPOs disclose their financial status, especially but not exclusively through those organizations' annual reports. Successfulness refers to the ways that NPOs present themselves as highly polished, high-impact professional organizations that are succeeding or will succeed in accomplishing their goals. And narrative virtuosity refers to the ability to tell a compelling story that will ultimately appeal not only to donors but also to donors' peers who might hear NPO stories and associate the stories with the donors. Transparency, successfulness, and narrative virtuosity establish relationships between philanthropists and NPOs in terms of relationships between philanthropic donations and NPO stories.

As is discussed below, classic anthropological scholarship quips that "there is no such thing as a free gift." In my analysis, one of the primary things that philanthropists eventually receive in return for their donations is an ethical connection to NPO stories. And transparency, successfulness, and narrative virtuosity are key aspects of how NPOs demonstrate to potential philanthropists that their stories are the sorts of ethical, effective ones with which donors would want to be associated.

Key Concepts: Economic Values, Audience, and Circulation

Economic value can be broadly defined as "the degree to which [things] are desired, particularly, as measured by how much others are willing to give up to get them" (Graeber 2001: 1; see also Cavanaugh and Shankar 2014: 53). While this is a core topic in the field of economics, anthropologists have long held views on the subject that diverge from those of economists.

One point of contention is the origin of capitalist monetary value. Economics texts tend to base theories of capitalism on the assumption that barter (disinterested exchange of one good for another) predated the invention of money. Anthropologists counter that there is no archaeological or ethnographic evidence to support such an assumption (Graeber 2011: ch. 2). Rather, anthropologists point to economies rooted in gift giving as the key to understanding economic values. This is especially significant for understanding contemporary global health because philanthropic donations are often described as gifts.

Indeed, anthropological evidence demonstrates that gift economies predate the introduction of money and continue to co-exist even within capitalist economies (e.g., Hutchinson 1992). The predominance of gift giving rather than barter makes sense if one considers that most pre-capitalist exchange happened between neighbors and kin rather than strangers (Graeber 2011: ch. 2). In gift exchange, gifts initiate and sustain long-term social activities of reciprocity that are shaped by clear if often implicit values and conventions (Mauss 2000 [1950]). People do not often insist on an immediate return when providing something to a family member, neighbor, or friend. Instead, they expect that they will receive something in turn when the time is right, relying on a set of shared cultural values that provide obligations and recommendations to the receiver of the gift. This is quite different from barter, where there is an immediate return and an explicit calculation of the value of the goods exchanged.

Anthropologists add that gift giving also plays a significant role in capitalist economies, because "capitalist commodity value is everywhere created through tapping and transforming non-capitalist social relations" (Tsing 2013: 21). In this context, it has been argued that commodification does symbolic violence to the sociality of gift giving, because the creation of a commodity occurs through the stripping of social connections from the item in question (Faudree 2020 on semiotic stripping; Agha 2011).

A significant part of contemporary global health NPO funding is derived from philanthropy, and this is often simply articulated as "giving." However, anthropological understandings of gift giving, commodification, and the socioeconomics of philanthropy complicate this notion. In many configurations of global health, philanthropists give not to aid recipients directly but to NPOs. This raises the question: what sort of long-term social activities of reciprocity are initiated through such gifts? My analysis in this chapter points toward the idea that rather than an eventual return on their donations, philanthropists become associated with the stories told by global health professionals and in particular become connected to the ethical values espoused in those stories (discussed further in Chapter 7). In the context of global capitalism, this type of philanthropy is a reversal of commodification. Whereas commodification strips social values, philanthropy semiotically laminates social meanings onto the transfer of money or other commodities (e.g., pharmaceutical drugs). And this lamination occurs through the circulation of stories.

Here, circulation refers to the ways that linguistic and communicative patterns are recontextualized—and their meaning thus transformed—as they circulate by being told to different audiences across different contexts (Goodwin and Duranti 1992; Briggs and Bauman 1992; Gal 2018). In one sense, it may seem strange to talk about words or stories circulating. After all, it is storytellers, audiences, recordings, and written representations of stories that actually move through the world; yet as one traces a word, a phrase, or a plot being retold across context and across storytellers, ideas move through the world and are transformed as they move, shaping storytelling participants' imagination about what was, is, or may be. In this process, audiences play a significant role in co-creating meaning regardless of whether they are active, passive, or imagined co-tellers (as in the case of recorded or broadcast stories) (Duranti 1986; Avineri 2021; Bell and Gibson 2011). Performers may change how they speak depending on who is in the audience, and these changes may shift the meaning of the stories (Bauman 1986; see also Bell 1984). The audience is a co-author, regardless of whether or not they actually speak (Duranti 1986).

The ways that audiences shape meaning depend in part on the relative power or authority of audiences and speakers (Inoue 2003). For instance, scholarship on race, power, and audience in the United States argues that the "white listening subject" may "dictate what is considered to be appropriate or correct (or alternatively, deficient or deviant) based on normative practices" (Avineri 2021: 4; see Flores and Rosa 2015). This matches what I found in my past research on global health, where real and imagined audiences of predominantly White global health researchers and aid workers shaped the ways that Black South African patient-activists created performances and told stories (Black 2019). Power dynamics thus impact how—and whether—(health) stories, performances, and phrases circulate (Briggs 2017; Briggs and Mantini-Briggs 2016). In this chapter, I examine how powerful audiences of philanthropists and donor corporations shape the stories that global health professionals tell, leading NPOs to focus on the three core values introduced above: transparency, successfulness, and narrative virtuosity.

Transparency

Transparency is a significant evaluative concept for global health, but also for all contemporary non-profit management and funding more generally. Its use is rooted in a belief that openly communicating about spending and donations will alleviate ethical issues. The term is used in at least three ways. First, transparency is sometimes linked to concerns about accountability and used to evaluate whether leaders in low- and middle-income countries are acting in ways that are corrupt. While this usage reflects some of the realities of how resource distribution may occur in contexts of scarcity, it also deploys racialized affect, shaping how people from high-income countries think about corruption (e.g., erroneously thinking of corruption as something that only or primarily happens in low- and middle-income countries). Second, transparency is sometimes used to describe the ways that health professionals from high-income countries could or should share information—both medical knowledge and the details of how interventions are being structured—with doctors, health professionals, and bureaucrats of low- and middle-income countries, enabling agency and autonomy among recipients of this information. Third, transparency is sometimes used to argue that private foundations and NPOs in high-income countries should report their financial information publicly (Sridhar and Batniji 2008). It is this third interpretation of transparency that I have found most often on display in public-facing communication of global health NPOs of the global North.

Global health organizations perform this version of transparency primarily through their websites—in particular, through yearly reports posted on these websites. This was first brought to my attention by a group of five undergraduate students (Kristina Ellis, Kate Leek, Scarlett Mayoralgo, Anna Rodriguez, and Savannah Setter) who worked with me to qualitatively code and analyze the key themes they found on six global health websites.[1] In that work, "transparency" was a key code/theme. While interpretive work was sometimes necessary to tag part of a webpage with this code, more often student researchers found it to be obvious. For instance, the Joint United Nations Programme on HIV/AIDS (UNAIDS) website includes a page titled "Transparency portal." The portal has links to a list of UNAIDS top contributors and to another page describing the "international aid transparency initiative."[2]

Similarly, a now-outdated version of the Task Force for Global Health website included a page titled "Financials," which featured a range of information—from internal revenue service (IRS) forms to the Task Force's conflict of interest policy and bylaws, along with a yearly consolidated audit report. The bottom of the page also shared the following statement:

> The Task Force for Global Health meets all 20 Charity Standards established by the Better Business Bureau. The Task Force is also certified by TRACE, an organization founded to assure partners and governments that international service agencies understand and comply with anti-bribery regulations. The Task Force meets all standards for certification. The Task Force has the highest level of transparency at

GuideStar, an information service that specializes in reporting on US non-profit companies.

This statement led me to investigate Guidestar. Guidestar is an organization—which has now been rebranded as "Candid" and referred to here as Candid—that mediates the relationship between NPOs, donors, and other "partners," by evaluating the transparency of NPOs and providing an evaluative list of them to potential donors and partners. Candid advertises to NPOs. For instance, on the organization's website, there is a link that an NPO can click to start the process of earning a Candid Seal of Transparency. The link text tells NPOs to "attract donors with your nonprofit profile," in order to "Earn a Seal of Transparency to give donors the information they need to support you."[3]

The fact that an organization such as Candid even exists is itself an indication of the significance of transparency as a value for contemporary NPO fundraising and planning purposes. The concept of transparency provides guidance to NPOs about what sorts of communicative actions should be taken, especially what sorts of information should be made available (publicly and/or to donors and partners); and over time, a set of multimodal poetic conventions, loosely shared among global health professionals, has developed for how to display their transparency to others (discussed below).

How to Obtain Platinum Transparency

On the subject of what sorts of actions to take and information to make available, Guidestar (which merged with Foundation Directory in 2019 and is now called Candid) helpfully (and transparently) posted a document online that defines what it takes to earn a bronze, silver, gold, and platinum transparency seal (Figure 4.1).[4]

This is just one organization's definition and system of evaluation of transparency. However, by 2021 this system had been utilized by over 75,000 organizations (about five percent of NPOs registered with the IRS). Almost all of these seal holders were public charities, two-thirds of which received over half of their revenue from donations (Koob and Brouwer 2021).[5] In addition to the Task Force, badge holders in 2023 included the Bill and Melinda Gates Foundation (which displayed a silver badge) and CARE (Cooperative for Assistance and Relief Everywhere) (which displayed a platinum badge).

The actions required to earn a bronze seal are fairly routine. An NPO is simply supposed to "provide basic information to make sure donors find you." Organizations are asked to provide a name and employer identification number (for the IRS), a mailing address, a website URL, a contact

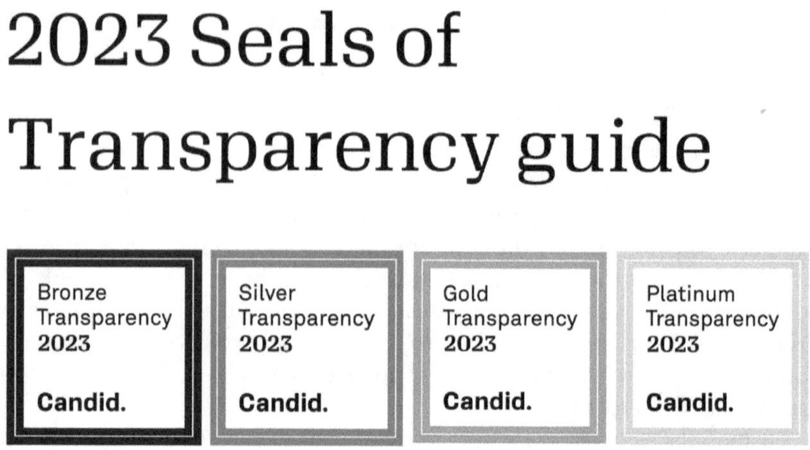

Figure 4.1 Seals of Transparency.

person and email, an organization leader's name, and a mission statement. To earn a silver seal, Candid asks NPOs to also "share program(s) information and brand details to guide funding decisions." This includes a logo, tagline, and social media usernames, as well as an answer to the question of whether or not the organization makes its own grants or donations to others. The silver seal also requires information about the NPO's programs such as target population, geographic area served, and program name, information, and description.

The gold seal asks for more detailed disclosures of the sorts that prompted my 2018 research team to notice transparency as a theme on global health websites. The list of required financial data includes either a recent audited financial statement or a laundry list of items: fiscal year start and end date, contributions/gifts/grants, total revenue, program expenses, administration expenses, total expenses, total assets, total liabilities, and net assets or fund balance. Gold seal certification also asks for leader demographics—race/ethnicity, gender identity, sexual orientation, and disability status—but this is not much of a requirement as an NPO can alternatively "decline to state." Finally, to earn a platinum seal, an organization must also share their strategic plan, as well as progress and results of that plan. This includes quantitative metrics of "success" (more on successfulness below).

The purpose of all this communicative work, as stated by Candid in its message to NPOs, is "to highlight your impact and boost your funding." While transparency could be interpreted as an epistemic or ethical value, here it is framed as an economic one. Or more precisely, there may be both ethical and economic values associated with transparency. The ethical value focuses on whether an NPO is spending the bulk of their money on their programs, supporting marginalized communities, and doing good. The economic value is based on how these actions are communicated to others, especially to potential donors.

Multimodal Poetics of Transparency

In addition to the Wellstar badges, NPOs communicate transparency through a set of multimodal semiotic conventions that appear across a range of documents and media. Nowhere are these more clearly on display than in NPOs' annual reports. The annual reports of two Atlanta-area organizations—the CDC Foundation and CARE—provide excellent examples of these conventions in action.[6] The CDC Foundation's downloadable report is titled "DonorReport_FactSheet" (a fairly clear indication of one of the report's intended audiences). One thing that these NPOs' annual reports share in common is their use of infographics, especially world maps (showing where NPOs work and how many people they serve), as well as charts that combine simple graphic icons with metrics and short verbal descriptions. In the CDC Foundation document (see Figure 4.2), for instance,

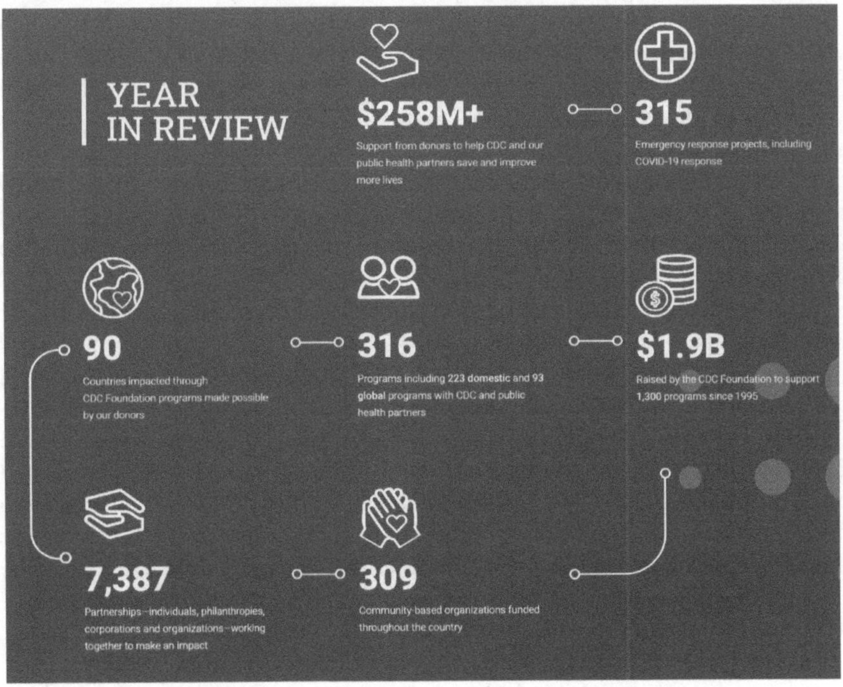

Figure 4.2 CDC Foundation Year in Review Infographic.

an infographic appears as their "year in review," while in the CARE document the infographic is titled "2021 CARE by the numbers." Both are focused on enumerating each foundation's successes.

The simplicity and clarity of the icons, numbers, and noun phrases of the CDC Foundation infographic provide donors—and potential donors—with the building blocks of a story that they can tell themselves and/or others about the NPO's work; and these plot points also serve as a confirmation of the good that donors have done. Four of these seven icons are accompanied by verb phrases in the passive voice: the object of an action has become the subject of the sentence (e.g., 309 community-based organizations funded throughout the country"). In many English-language contexts, passive voice constructions are agent-less and these phrases are sometimes used to avoid assigning responsibility or blame (Duranti 2004: 465–466). One effect of using passive voice might be to de-emphasize the NPO's role and instead make it possible for donors to see themselves as aiding in these accomplishments, though the NPO's role is implied by the appearance of these phrases in the yearly report of the NPO.

Another effect of these passive voice constructions is that they make it possible to make statements that start with numbers, a pattern that also occurs in other organizations' reports. For instance, the globe icon and its accompanying phrase accomplishes a range of semiotic work through a compact message: "90 countries impacted through CDC Foundation programs made possible by our donors." Here, "impact," which is a key term in successfulness (to be discussed below), is used. The NPO is also mentioned, and donors are recognized as an underlying force behind the CDC Foundation programs. Enumeration and passive voice allow for all of the statements to parallel the grammar of the funding report ($258 million plus "support from donors to help CDC..."), while also providing rhetorical appeal.

Another feature that yearly reports often share in common is a list of donors and partners sorted into groups according to the amount of money that they donated. For instance, the CARE donors and partners list has a category for those who have given over one million dollars in "cumulative lifetime giving," down to those who have given between 10,000 and 25,000 dollars—those giving less than 10,000 dollars are not mentioned in the annual report. The CDC Foundation, on the other hand, has an exhaustive list online of all donors down to $25. That list has so many people that it would be inconvenient to include in a PDF or printed report.[7] The organization thus helpfully tells donors, "You can use the 'Search All Donors' button at the top to find your name in the report."

I asked a philanthropist who I know—a person who does significant volunteer work with NPOs and also donates money to NPOs—about these donor lists. If people do not want credit for their donations, as they sometimes claim, why would these lists exist? I expected the answer to be something cynical. Do people do secretly want credit? Are they really expecting social gain for their donations? While not ruling these possibilities out, my contact described a personal experience of being asked to be named as a donor despite his expressed desire to stay anonymous. When he asked the NPO's leader why they needed to do this, the leader explained that naming him (the donor) was an important way for the NPO to provide an example to other potential donors. Indeed, my contact added, one purpose of donor lists is to exert peer pressure. If most of the people in one's elite social circle are donating to a particular cause, one does not want to be seen as the only one to not donate. Like other aspects of transparency, then, donor lists are at least in part about soliciting other donations.

For donors, though, it is important to note that transparency does have an ethical dimension. People who donate want to know that their money is not being wasted and that it is being primarily spent on communities in need rather than enriching NPO employees. Evidence such as Candid's "Seals of Transparency" document indicates the economic value of transparency for attracting and retaining donors. Through the communicative actions associated with transparency, especially through donor lists, the ethical values of global health may be semiotically laminated onto philanthropists' public personas.

Successfulness

Successfulness is another value that shapes the economics of global health. This term does not refer to the actual successes of an organization's health interventions (though those are important). Rather, successfulness is about the semiotics of success—the ways that a high production value in the aesthetics of NPO media design communicates the idea that an organization is or could be successful. Across social contexts in the United States and elsewhere, high production value may function as a powerful index of prestige and social value (Meek and Messing 2007). In global health, this valence intersects with donors' desire to contribute to and be associated with efforts that are successful—and to not have their money go to waste. One key term for successfulness is effectiveness: to be effective is one important way to be successful. Another key term is impact, which refers to how an organization significantly affects or influences some sector of global health, often expressed through metrics and stories about the lives of beneficiaries of global health interventions.

Success was another a theme that communications specialist Scott raised in our interview (discussed at the beginning of the chapter).

There, Scott explained to me that *demonstrations* of success shape how global health stories are told and which stories are chosen to be told. He used the term "success stories" to understand his organization's public-facing communication, describing such stories as a part of how his organization could demonstrate its impact to donors:

Excerpt 10: Be Meaningful to a Potential Donor (starting at 4 min 8 sec)

> Scott: We really wanted to demonstrate our impact on global health with the idea that that will be meaningful to a potential donor. So "what are you doing to move the needle?" So, we built our success stories around our work... That has taken many forms, we've had case studies—you might have seen some of the case studies we've developed on the website? We also have been trying to pull in human interest stories to humanize the impact of our work at the individual level.

Though it is a common enough phrase to have been said without much thought, it is perhaps indicative of global health's general fixation on metrics that Scott uses the idiom "move the needle" (a metaphor based on the image of a measuring instrument with a pointer or needle) to refer to storytelling that otherwise seems to be focused on the individual and the qualitative. He describes case studies and human-interest stories as demonstrations of impact—success stories—aimed at potential donors.

Finally, Scott concludes his discussion with an explicit turn to measurement and metrics:

Excerpt 11: Metrics to Evaluate Our Impact (starting at 4 min 51 sec)

> Scott: Also looking at metrics to evaluate our impact. For many years we evaluated our impact by the number of treatments of drugs we shipped, but that wasn't—again, it's not very meaningful; those are metrics that are meaningful to [the pharmaceutical company] but not meaningful to an external audience. So we try to translate that into the number of people who we have served in a particular year through our partners. So, we've come up with a variety of different metrics that we track every year and that informs the content of the website and our other communications channels.

Here, Scott provides an explanation of the sorts of enumeration that is prominent in NPOs' yearly reports, describing a complex process of "translation" through which quantitative measures of pharmaceutical drugs shipped are transformed into quantitative measures of the number of people served. Notably, the actual serving of people occurs "through our partners." As discussed in Chapter 3, this phrase holds much hidden meaning. Using this term that holds ethical value, Scott enables the NPO to lay claim to the impact of health interventions despite not being the ones providing hands on care to target populations. Scott sums things up by noting that the number of people served and other metrics are utilized on the website and other communications channels. In other words, these measures of impact are turned into stories.

The Shape of Human-Interest Stories

Scott's description matches the human-interest stories that I have analyzed that come from global health NPO annual reports. In three of these reports—published by the CDC Foundation, CHAMPS (Child Health and Mortality Prevention Surveillance) Health,[8] and CARE—human-interest stories appear alongside enumerations of impact. The website version of the CDC Foundation report includes nine videos of health professionals speaking about their work (titled "voices of impact"), below which photos appear along with links to eight "impact stories." Similarly, a CARE infographic that mentions 1,495 projects in 102 countries serving one hundred million people appears just before a section of the organization's annual report titled "stories of impact."

These stories, which are situated near infographics, are aligned with the two organizations' core strategies. The CARE website describes the organization as working to "save lives, defeat poverty, and achieve social justice." And the NPO's annual report features stories about food and water, crisis response, climate, education, and equality. These foci feature quotations from beneficiaries of CARE programs. For instance, a blurb titled "Fighting malnutrition one village at a time" describes Souadé Aboubacar: she is a mother of nine from rural Niger who is participating in Hamzari, which is "a five year, $33 million CARE program (in partnership with USAID) that addresses food insecurity and malnutrition." Aboubacar explains, "Before Hamzari, we did not know about enriched porridge and bean purree… we noticed that by eating this porridge and bean puree our children are in good health and grow normally, without diarrhea or signs of malnutrition." This impact story makes it seem as if the primary function of the Hamzari program is to educate impoverished people about proper nutrition. However, the program is actually much larger—it includes five other NPOs plus unnamed "technical partners" and addresses agriculture, livestock, farmer-managed natural regeneration of land, nutrition and health, and hygiene.[9] Despite this, the Hamzari impact story in the donor report does not describe most of these complexities of the program.

It simply gives readers a sense that their donation is doing something good for poor people in Africa as represented by particular individuals and their stories. In this way, the individualized aid-recipient story reproduces liable and empowering affect (as described in Chapter 3).

Some organizations' human-interest stories do not rely on individual care recipients as "poster-children" for the organizations. Rather, the stories focus on the overall shape and significance of the organizations' interventions. This difference is likely connected to the distinct donor audiences for each organization. CHAMPS Health, which is primarily funded by the Gates Foundation, has an annual report that is technical, science-oriented, and focuses on the preliminary findings of the program. The CDC Foundation, which caters to donors likely to want to support public health (including but not limited to current and former CDC employees), focuses on the overall shape of its ongoing public health programs.

CHAMPS Health is far more techno-optimistic in its approach than CARE. Its human-interest stories are featured in a section of its annual report titled "Building trust through community engagement." The feature story describes how CHAMPS is using theater and radio to communicate scientific medical information. For instance,

> In Kersa and Harar, Ethiopia, CHAMPS uses participatory community theater to deliver information about child and maternal health, help explain our work and share CHAMPS results. Actors are recruited from the same communities where they perform and help adapt scripts to ensure that the show addresses community needs in an authentic, engaging way. These performances have increased community acceptance of CHAMPS.

As described in this story, this participatory community theater program is designed according to the culture-as-barrier to scientific medicine model described earlier in this book. CHAMPS is using theater to overcome a perceived barrier to their science-based intervention—a barrier supposedly posed by Ethiopian culture that can be overcome through culturally relevant education. It is notable that this theatrical performance is described as addressing community needs. To which community needs is CHAMPS referring? The need to be educated about CHAMPS? This seems like a strange way of framing needs in a context where CHAMPS is collecting tissue samples from recently deceased children and where the causes of death identified by the NPO include treatable illnesses such as malnutrition, tuberculosis, and malaria. This version of "community needs" makes sense when one assumes a techno-optimistic evaluative framework in which CHAMPS' efforts to scientifically model child mortality will lead to better health interventions in the future, such that community acceptance of CHAMPS is a necessary step along the way.

Art, performance, and music are indeed crucial tools for community-engaged work. I learned this in my previous research in South Africa (in 2008) with a Zulu gospel choir that was an HIV support group, AIDS activist organization, and performance troupe (Black 2019; see also Barz 2006). However, in the case of the choir with which I worked, group members received extensive training about scientific models of HIV/AIDS treatment and prevention, then they took the lead in identifying key themes and issues that were relevant to them and their home communities, then writing and performing songs. Arts-based interventions should treat community-based performers as co-designers and authors from the earliest stages of a program, rather than simply as the means to the end of communicating what global health organizations from high-income countries deem to be significant.

Like CHAMPS Health, the CDC Foundation also reports that they are using the arts to address vaccine skepticism and "communicate accurate public health information." As this NPO works primarily with public health agencies in the United States and abroad, its stories focus on the broad contours of health programs. For instance, the first story in its report is titled "Improving water, sanitation and hygiene to fight disease." This appears alongside a picture of a Black African woman, who is wearing a hijab, surgical mask, and latex gloves, taking a water sample from a tap at an outside sink. It is important to note that this featuring of a global health professional who is a PERSON OF COLOR is a welcome counterpoint to some of the other discussed examples of racialized affect. The text of this impact story reads:

> Globally, gaps in basic water, sanitation and hygiene (WASH) services in healthcare facilities place approximately 1.8 billion people at heightened risk of diseases. With support from the Conrad N. Hilton Foundation, Wallace Genetic Foundation and World Vision Inc., the CDC Foundation is engaged in three major projects to improve WASH infrastructure and waste management in healthcare facilities. Partnering with implementing organizations and local governments in Burkina Faso, Ethiopia, Ghana, Niger and Uganda, the CDC Foundation is working with CDC to assess and track progress toward national and global standards for WASH in healthcare facilities, increase uptake of WASH practices and provide technical assistance to partners. Through this vital work, the CDC Foundation and our partners are ensuring healthcare facilities in high-priority settings are implementing evidence-based, field-tested best practices to reduce the burden of infectious diseases and save lives.

This story is about a topic that could lend itself to structural interventions (water, sanitation, and hygiene), yet the narrative nonetheless emphasizes a techno-optimistic approach, using many of the building blocks of techno-optimistic plots that will be discussed in depth in the next chapter. First, there is a statement of a biomedicalized problem: gaps in WASH services place people at heightened risk of diseases. There is a discussion of what the organization is doing, saying that the NPO (supported by large donors) is improving WASH infrastructure and waste management in healthcare facilities. There is a mention of partners, invoking ethical values. And there is an imagined hopeful future where there is to be a reduction in the burden of infectious diseases. This human-interest story is quite ingenious, in the sense that the CDC Foundation has crafted a compelling success story in which the CDC Foundation is not directly providing care. Rather, it is assessing, tracking progress, increasing uptake of practices, and providing technical assistance. Just as communications specialist Scott talked about "translating" the number of drugs donated into the number of people served, this story translates technical assistance to partners into saving lives.

Another CDC Foundation impact story, titled "Supporting American Indian Elders During COVID-19," features quotations from the leader of an NPO partner organization that itself "provided critically needed medical supplies to seven local partner organizations across four tribal communities."[10] Again, the CDC Foundation manages to turn indirect action (working with a partner who is working with their own partners) into a compelling story. While the intervention described in this story is not aimed at changing structural conditions, it also is not explicitly techno-optimistic. Instead, it focuses on providing basic supplies such as personal protective equipment and essential items such as hygiene kits, walkers, and wheelchairs, and mattresses that would enable elders to safely isolate in cabins built for the purpose of isolation during COVID-19 surges. Still, given the general aims of CDC and global health NPOs during the pandemic (discussed in detail in Chapter 5), it is likely that an underlying premise of this initiative was to keep elders safe until a vaccine had been developed. Along with the written story, this part of the annual report includes images of two tribal elders wearing surgical masks and an image of boxes of what are presumably medical supplies.

As communications specialist Scott suggested, these and other human-interest stories found in global health NPOs' annual reports provide indicators of an NPO's impact in a way that may be appealing to past and future donors. The reports also appear in glossy printed format in many NPO offices and are ready to be showcased as evidence of an NPO's past successes and ability to be successful. Many annual report stories are techno-optimistic in nature. These narratives are emplotted in ways that linked past technologically-based actions of the NPO to health improvements in the present or present actions to imagined health improvements in the future. And the narratives utilize configurations of multimodal poetics—including the high production value of high-resolution images of aid recipients and health workers, as well as carefully designed color-coordinated fonts, backgrounds, and infographics. Together, these storytelling features evoke successfulness, which is the idea or feeling of being successful. This idea/feeling is an economic value in the sense that it is meant to enhance the circulation of stories about an NPO among existing donors and potential donors. Successfulness encourages monetary donations, thereby establishing relationships between NPOs and philanthropists.

Narrative Virtuosity

In the context of global health, I use the term narrative virtuosity to refer to NPO leaders' abilities to deftly craft compelling stories. Across many cultural contexts, virtuosity is an important component of some but not all genres of performance. For instance, jazz musicians highly value the cultivation of incredible improvisational and performance skill (Day 2000). In contrast, in Indie music what is most valued is musicians' ability to perform in ways that are deemed to be authentic (real or sincere), and virtuosity is described as a barrier to that authentic expression (Fonarow 2006). Still, in many contexts virtuosic displays are valued parts of performance genres (Bauman 2011). At first glance, public discourses associated with global health seem to better fit a model in which virtuosity is downplayed or dismissed. After all (as will be discussed in Chapter 5), knowledge production in science is thought of as distinct from the concerns of verbal aesthetics. The truth of science is not supposed to be dependent on one's ability to communicate it. Just as global health professionals' public speaking is not always at first glance identifiable as storytelling, their prowess as storytellers is not always clearly or explicitly valued. However, a closer look reveals that narrative virtuosity is of existential significance to the field.

I first became aware of the value of narrative virtuosity while quarantining with a possible COVID-19 infection early in the pandemic in March 2020. At that time, I happened upon a prescient documentary series, "Pandemic: How to Prevent an Outbreak." Episode one of the series provides a view of the inner workings of a biotech company named Distributed Bio. In the film, the company is developing a universal flu vaccine—one that would prevent all possible mutations of the flu virus. The documentary shows a presentation by Jake Glanville, the co-founder, chief scientific officer, and chairperson of Distributed Bio. Glanville speaks about the efforts of his company at a conference for therapeutic discovery in New York. In a voice-over interview interwoven with audio-video of his presentation, Glanville explains that he used to get stage fright before such conferences. However, he says that he had to become "an effective communicator," continuing, "if I wasn't able to communicate my science, then it was almost like the science didn't exist." Glanville connects his particular interest in communication with storytelling. He indicates that he cannot simply communicate his scientific results in scholarly journals; rather, he wants to be a "really good" storyteller. One of Glanville's stated goals as chairperson is to attract investors who will financially support his vision due to their belief in the company's long-term profitability. This would be realized if the company's vaccine were developed and sold to healthcare providers, generating profits that would enrich the company's investors. To do so, though, Glanville must be given his chance; and whether or not he is given that chance (through financial investment) depends in part on whether or not he tells a good story.

Glanville explains how he thinks about performing in front of audiences of scientists and potential investors (beginning at 14 min 04 sec in the documentary):

> I never memorize a specific speech. I think about the arc of the story I'm going to tell, and really good storytelling, those rules apply to science. It's basically the same rules that our ancestors did around the campfire, right? First you have to introduce the terrible monster. In this case it's influenza... We have created these amazing vaccine technologies that are arguably the greatest advances since sanitation and fire, and yet they don't work on rapidly mutating viruses like the flu, for instance... Then you present the hero. That there's some new technology that exists that could potentially create a breakthrough.

Here, Glanville focuses especially on the emplotment of techno-optimism: pathogens are the monsters, and novel scientific technologies are the heroes of his stories. And he explains that his goal is "really good storytelling"—in other words, narrative virtuosity. In the documentary film, Distributed Bio, which is a for-profit company, is looking for investors hoping to receive financial gain in exchange for their contributions. NPOs, on the other hand, must find donors. Still, the value of narrative virtuosity remains similarly significant, if often implicit, for the structuring of storytelling performances in order to attract donors.

Folk Hero Bill Foege and the Importance of Narrativized Goals

Bill Foege, according to at least one Decatur-based NPO, is a "folk hero." This is the description of Foege provided by MAP International, an organization associated with Christian missionary medicine, which has a series of awards named the Bill Foege Health Awards (2022 sponsors included Delta airlines, Emory University, and the CDC Foundation).[11] Recall that Foege enjoyed a long and illustrious career in global health (described in Chapter 2).

His career is particularly powerful given the fact that it has been combined with his storytelling prowess.

The exchange recounted here happened at the September 2015 event hosted by the Task Force for Global Health to celebrate the NPO's 30th anniversary (also discussed in Chapter 3). Recall that this event featured a panel discussion with Foege and other global health luminaries. During that discussion, Jim Kim (then-president of the World Bank) provided comments about Bill Foege's storytelling in the midst of his own story.

Moderator Mark Rosenberg has just finished introducing all of the roundtable participants (which include Paul Farmer, Bill Foege, Jim Yong Kim, and Matshidiso Moeti), questionably deploying the concept of accompaniment. He then turns to Jim Kim and asks about the connection between poverty and disease, focusing on Kim's recent World Bank announcement that for the first time the percentage of people living in poverty in the world would likely fall to under ten percent.[12]

Kim notes that the past fifteen years has indeed seen a rapid drop in the number of people living in extreme poverty, but that this is mostly due to high rates of economic growth in China. But as he is about to launch into an extended narrative about his work at the World Bank, Kim abruptly shifts his focus to Bill Foege.

"Now, but I have to go back and talk about Bill a little bit." Jim Kim smiles and laughs. Audience members laugh with him.

Bill Foege humorously interjects, "You don't have to," and the audience laughs louder.

"I do," Kim retorts. "So, first of all, I just want to say that, you know—and I can say this with all honesty—I would not be here today without the support of Bill Foege." Kim mentions the grant that he and Paul Farmer received from the Gates Foundation, calling that grant "transformative." He credits Foege and Rosenberg with convincing the Gates Foundation to provide that grant.

Kim continues, "The way I think about just about everything is affected by the stories I heard from Bill, especially about the 1984 meeting, and about what it meant to set a goal." While he does not explain to what 1984 refers, Kim is talking about the 1984 meeting in Italy when the Task Force (then newly formed and called the Task Force for Child Survival), the Rockefeller Foundation, UNICEF, and others created the goal of raising low childhood immunization rates in low-income countries—the result of which would be called the child survival resolution (discussed in Chapter 2). It is notable that Kim specifically mentions stories here, indicating that there is something special about Foege's storytelling.

Kim then says that he followed Foege's example to set the "most outrageous target anyone could have imagined" for reducing poverty in the early 2000s, explaining, "but you know, the importance of a target is that it has to force you to change the way you do your work." In global health, Kim insists, targets are a way to orient the actions of a group toward a common goal (e.g., reducing poverty or decreasing child mortality). I would add that targets are also incipient stories that connect past and current actions with projected outcomes through emplotment.

Kim goes on to tell a story about the importance of targets for World Bank initiatives, discussing the target to end extreme poverty by 2030 and the target to provide universal access to financial services by 2020. He says that he was prompted by his team at the World Bank to announce the 2020 target during a panel, and so he did so. But then:

Excerpt 12: What's the Plan? (starting at 29 min 52 sec)

> Jim Kim: after the meeting I came back [to my team] and I said, "okay. So what's the plan?" and they said "um, we don't have a plan." ((audience laughs)). And I said, "so why did you make me do—" "oh, we know you love targets and you love end dates." ((audience laughs)). So I said, "okay, tomorrow I want you to set up a war room, I want you to have dedicated people doing it, and give me a plan," for universal access to financial services. And after about a year, they came up with one. And last year, we were able to announce that we think we can get a billion people access to financial services, MasterCard and Visa said, "and we'll take 500 million each."

This story is not directly about health care, but it is told in the context of a discussion about the connections between poverty and disease during a Task Force for Global Health panel discussion. Similar to Bill Foege's stories, Kim's telling elicits audience laughter while driving home his point (in this case, a point about the relationship between targets and organizational action). And this story is about a targeted, techno-optimistic intervention involving partnership between a multilateral institution and private companies who donate to a cause.

As he finishes this story, Kim turns his head and looks at Bill Foege, then reaches over and puts his hand on Foege's arm.

Kim concludes,

> So, everything I do, Bill, everything I do, is impacted by your career. And also—whenever I give advice, I always tell Bill Foege stories. And so, one of the great lines that you've heard many many times is that no one will follow the call of an uncertain trumpet. That's a great one.

Notably (in the context of the Christian underpinnings of early global health), the idea of an uncertain trumpet not being a good way to lead forces into battle is mentioned in the Bible. However, this is also an excellent metaphor for the economic value of narrative virtuosity in global health. A strong trumpet calls troops to action. And virtuosic storytelling aligns donors, institutions, and global health professionals with specific narratives and narrativized goals, attracting funding and imagining the possibility of positive intervention outcomes into being.

Conclusion

On July 12, 2008, in Atlanta, CDC hosted a reunion for people who had worked on the Smallpox Eradication Program (SEP) in Southeast Asia and East Africa. A video of the program, titled "Smallpox Eradication in India, Bangladesh, and Somalia: Living History, Lessons Learned, Celebration," includes a presentation by the seemingly ever-present and illustrious Dr. William Foege.[13]

A recording of the reunion shows a moderator sitting at the kind of table one might see at any academic conference, with a tablecloth and skirt, a pitcher and glasses of water for speakers, and microphones connected to a set of speakers. He speaks to an auditorium full of people. The moderator announces Foege, explaining that Foege is going to talk about what smallpox eradication contributes to the future of global health. In other words, Foege will present an imaginative vision of the future based on the lessons he learned as one of the key players in the SEP. The moderator cedes the floor to Foege, who is standing at a nearby podium in front of CDC flags. Bill Foege's talk is inspirational and wide-ranging. He calls the 20th century as the century of physics and the 21st century as the century of biology, arguing that the great scientific discoveries of this century will come from biology.

Nine minutes into his speech, Foege asks himself a question: "What's the biggest change from my perspective in what will happen in global health?" Then he answers himself:

Excerpt 13: 21st-Century Challenges (Starting at 9 min 0 sec)

> Foege: Global health people will stop thinking like poor people. In the past we've always thought we didn't deserve more resources because we didn't get [them]. And so we always made do with what we had and we always had less than what we needed, and it <u>never</u> entered our minds, <u>never</u>, that some rich person might get interested in global health. And if we had ever thought of that, it never would have entered our minds that the richest couple in the <u>world</u> might get interested in global health. And if <u>that</u> had entered our minds, we never would have thought, "they'll get the next richest person also interested in global health" ((audience laughs)). And so this is going to make us think in a different way and be much bolder.

In his dry but playful style, Foege suggests that past global health efforts were underfunded. Health professionals learned to make things work with what they had available to them (the ethics of pragmatism). Foege's repeated emphasis on never (e.g., "it never entered our minds") is both a compelling rhetorical device and an indication that the shift to private philanthropic funding of global health has been surprising and unprecedented. As mentioned in Chapter 2, 2008 (when this event was held) was the burgeoning of what Foege accurately predicts to be a new era in global health—an era precipitated by huge novel sources of philanthropic funding from billionaires like Bill Gates, Mark Zuckerberg, and others.

Despite his prophetic accuracy, Foege does not anticipate some of the changes that will be precipitated by having the wealthiest people in the world interested in the field. How might priorities change as global health professionals re-orient their work to write grants and pitch projects in ways that can appeal to philanthropists? How might philanthropists thus exert undue influence over future interventions? Nor does Foege mention an issue of existential importance for NPOs: how can NPO professionals convince the wealthiest people to donate money to their particular organization rather than another?

The ethical values of global health in the global North certainly play a role in answering these questions. A record of effectiveness is important, as is a techno-optimistic orientation that showcases an NPO's projected ability to continue to be effective in ways that are in sync with the priorities of the world's best capitalists. Also important is the sense that an NPO collaborates with partners in low- and middle-income countries and helps those who are most in need (something that is often accomplished by employing racialized affect). But none of these things are relevant unless an NPO can communicate them to potential donors and thereby make an NPO's story circulate—as told to donors, by donors, and around those donors to others. Representatives of global health NPOs thus must also be skilled storytellers.

Together, the key values of transparency, successfulness, and narrative virtuosity shape how global health stories are told. These values are economic in the sense that they are oriented toward the potential to generate monetary contributions—contributions that, according to annual reports, websites, and global health professionals themselves, are linked with the circulation of stories. Transparency and successfulness suggest to philanthropists that donations will be well-spent, while narrative virtuosity helps stories to circulate, being told among global health professionals, to (potential) donors, and to others as a way to celebrate the contributions of donors and the work being accomplished.

These economic values are interconnected with the ethical values discussed in the previous chapter and the epistemic values to be discussed in Chapter 5. And crucially, these values end up shaping not only the stories that are told but also the interventions that are planned and carried out by NPOs of the global North. Techno-optimism and racialized affect dominate public-facing global health stories in part because these sorts of stories appeal to philanthro-capitalists. Such stories allow donors to feel that they are "doing well by doing good" (a phrase used by Scott during our interview) without interrogating the socioeconomic underpinnings of wealth creation in the global capitalist economy or the remnants of colonial institutions that still haunt global health today. This is not all bad. Global health professionals celebrate the flexibility and speed with which NPOs and public-private partnerships can respond to health emergencies, in contrast to the sometimes sloth-like movements of institutional bureaucracies and the political machinations associated with government-run programs. However, there is much room for improvement, particularly making changes to global health stories to de-emphasize racialized affect, complement techno-optimism with articulations of the need for structural change, and thus leave space for visions of the future that will help to decolonize of the field.

Notes

1 The six websites, accessed from September to December 2018, were the sites for the Africare, the Bill and Melinda Gates Foundation, Care, the Task Force for Global Health, UNAIDS, and the World Health Organization.
2 The current version of this webpage can be found here: https://open.unaids.org.
3 https://www.guidestar.org. Accessed 3/27/23.
4 This section is based on an analysis of this document, which can be found here: http://cdn.candid.org/images/nonprofit-profiles/seals/2023/candid-seals-guide-2023.pdf?_gl=1*hb3heb*_ga*MTMzNjI2ODY3NC4xNjc5OTIzOTEx*_ga_5W8PXYYGBX*MTY3OTkyMzkxMC4xLjEuMTY3OTkyNDUyNS42MC4wLjA.&_ga=2.21751032.2123813346.1679923912-1336268674.1679923911&_gac=1.94635630.1679923912.CjwKCAjw_YShBhAiEiwAMomsEG-kXUIiwaP14ciuGGf5JUCjGRsm-Ku0JEDmN6Ngjq2E3vKSgmkTd3xoCp8QQAvD_BwE. Accessed on 3/23/23.
5 https://blog.candid.org/post/a-look-at-organizations-that-have-earned-guidestar-seals-of-transparency/. Accessed 3/27/23.
6 https://www.cdcfoundation.org/FY2022/index.html. Accessed 3/29/2023, and https://www.care.org/news-and-stories/resources/care-usa-2021-annual-report/. Accessed 3/29/2023.
7 https://www.cdcfoundation.org/FY2022/donors?group=mahoney. Accessed 3/29/23.
8 https://champshealth.org/resources/champs-year-5-annual-report/. Accessed 4/19/23.
9 https://pdf.usaid.gov/pdf_docs/PA00X1NK.pdf. Accessed 4/19/23.
10 https://www.cdcfoundation.org/FY2022/supporting-american-indian-elders-during-covid.html. Accessed 3/23/2023.
11 https://www.map.org/bill-foege-global-health-awards/ Accessed 4/25/2023; MAP International has an office located across the street from the Task Force for Global Health.

12 https://www.youtube.com/watch?v=24YkghgecNo&t=1027s. Accessed 4/26/2023;beginning at 22 min 53 sec in the YouTube video.
13 "Foege: Disease Prevention," *The Global Health Chronicles*, https://globalhealthchronicles.org/items/show/3004. Accessed 3/14/2023.

References

Agha, Asif. 2011. "Commodity Registers." *Journal of Linguistic Anthropology* 21 (1): 22–53.

Avineri, Netta. 2021. "Audience (and Audience Design)." In *The International Encyclopedia of Linguistic Anthropology*, edited by James Stanslaw. John Wiley & Sons. https://doi.org/10.1002/9781118786093.iela0019

Barz, Gregory. 2006. *Singing for Life: HIV/AIDS and music in Uganda*. New York: Routledge.

Basilico, Matthew, Jonathan Weigel, Anjali Motgi, Jacob Bor, and Salmaan Keshavjee. 2013. "Health For All? Competing Theories and Geopolitics." In *Reimagining Global Health: An Introduction*, edited by Paul Farmer, Jim Yong Kim, Arthur Kleinman, and Matthew Basilico, 74–110. Berkeley: University of California Press.

Bauman, Richard. 1986. "'I Go Into More Detail Now to be Sure': Narrative Variation and the Shifting Contexts of Traditional Storytelling." In *Story, Performance, and Event*, 78–111. New York: Cambridge University Press.

Bauman, Richard. 2011. "Commentary: Foundations in Performance." *Journal of Sociolinguistics* 15 (5): 707–720.

Bell, Allan. 1984. "Language Style as Audience Design." *Language in Society* 13 (2): 145–204.

Bell, Allan, and Andy Gibson, eds. 2011. "Staging Language: An Introduction to the Sociolinguistics of Performance." *A Special Issue of the Journal of Sociolinguistics* 15(5).

Black, Steven P. 2019. *Speech and Song at the Margins of Global Health: Zulu Tradition, HIV Stigma, and AIDS Activism in South Africa*. New Brunswick, NJ: Rutgers University Press.

Briggs, Charles L. 2017. "Towards Communicative Justice in Health." *Medical Anthropology* 36 (4): 287–304.

Briggs, Charles L., and Richard Bauman. 1992. "Genre, Intertextuality, and Social Power." *Journal of Linguistic Anthropology* 2 (2): 131–172.

Briggs, Charles L., and Clara Mantini-Briggs. 2016. *Tell Me Why My Children Died: Rabies, Indigenous Knowledge, and Communicative Justice*. Durham, NC: Duke University.

Cavanaugh, Jillian R., and Shalini Shankar. 2014. "Producing Authenticity in Global Capitalism: Language, Materiality, and Value." *American Anthropologist* 116 (1): 51–64.

Day, William. 2000. "Knowing as Instancing: Jazz Improvisation and Moral Perfectionism." *The Journal of Aesthetics and Art Criticism* 58 (2): 100–111.

Duranti, Alessandro. 1986. "The Audience as Co-Author." *Text* 6 (3): 239–247.

Duranti, Alessandro. 2004. "Agency in language." In *A Companion to Linguistic Anthropology*, edited by Alessandro Duranti, 451–473. Malden, MA: Blackwell Publishing.

Faudree, Paja. 2020. "'Making Medicine' with *Salvia divinorum*: Competing Approaches and Their Implications." *Medical Anthropology* 39 (7): 582–596.

Flores, Nelson, and Jonathan Rosa. 2015. "Undoing Appropriateness: Raciolinguistic Ideologies and Language Diversity in Education." *Harvard Educational Review* 85 (2): 149–171.

Fonarow, Wendy. 2006. *Empire of Dirt: The Aesthetics and Rituals of British Indie Music*. Middletown, CT: Wesleyan University Press.

Gal, Susan. 2018. "Registers in Circulation: The Social Organization of Interdiscursivity." *Signs and Society* 6 (1): 1–24.

Goodwin, Charles, and Alessandro Duranti. 1992. "Rethinking Context: An Introduction." In *Rethinking Context: Language as an Interactive Phenomenon*, edited by Alessandro Duranti and Charles Goodwin, 1–42. New York: Cambridge University Press.

Graeber, David. 2001. *Toward an Anthropological Theory of Value: the False Coin of Our Own Dreams*. New York: Palgrave.

Graeber, David. 2011. *Debt: The First 5,000 Years*. Brooklyn, NY: Melville House Publishing.

Hutchinson, Sharon E. 1992. "The Cattle of Money and the Cattle of Girls among the Nuer, 1930–83." *American Ethnologist* 19 (2): 294–316.

Inoue, Miyako. 2003. "The Listening Subject of Japanese Modernity and His Auditory Double: Citing, Sighting, and Siting the Modern Japanese Woman." *Cultural Anthropology* 18 (2): 156–193.

Koob, Anna, and Carol Brouwer. 2021. "A Look at Organizations That Have Earned Guidestar Seals of Transparency." *Candid Blog*, April 13, 2021. https://blog.candid.org/post/a-look-at-organizations-that-have-earned-guidestar-seals-of-transparency/.

Mauss, Marcel. 2000 [1950]. *The Gift: The Form and Reason for Exchange in Archaic Societies*. Translated by W. D. Halls. New York: Norton.

Meek, Barbara A., and Jacqueline Messing. 2007. "Framing Indigenous Languages as Secondary to Matrix Languages." *Anthropology and Education Quarterly* 38 (2): 99–118.

Mei, Yuyang. 2017. "Neoliberal Optimism: Applying Market Techniques to Global Health." *Medical Anthropology* 36 (4): 381–395.

Sridhar, Devi, and Rajaie Batniji. 2008. "Misfinancing Global Health: A Case for Transparency in Disbursements and Decision Making." *The Lancet* 372 (9644): 1185–1191.

Tsing, Anna. 2013. "Sorting Out Commodities: How Capitalist Value Is Made Through Gifts." *HAU: Journal of Ethnographic Theory* 3 (1): 21–43.

5 The Emplotment of Epistemic Values

On March 12, 2020, on Twitter (now known as "X"), former president Barack Obama posted a "flatten-the-curve" graphic and Vox article explaining the concept—one that many people became familiar with during the COVID-19 pandemic (image not included due to copyright issues).[1] He wrote, "If you're wondering whether it's an overreaction to cancel large gatherings and public events (and I love basketball), here's a useful primer as to why these measures can slow the spread of the virus and save lives. We have to look out for each other." In the tidy poetics of this tweet, Obama pairs alliteration (*s*low the *s*pread of the viru*s* and *s*ave live*s*) with an ethical framework of obligation and responsibility invoked through the verb "have to" (we have to look out for each other). In doing so, he follows a well-established pattern of the use of wave graphics in scientific discourses about epidemics. Historian of science David S. Jones and anthropologist Stefan Helmreich (2020) explain the history of waves in epidemic discourses: "waves emerge first as a device of data visualization, then evolve into an object of mathematical modeling and causal investigation and finally morph into a tool of persuasion, intervention, and governance." The authors describe epidemic graphics as "combining math and morality, rational forecasting and affective persuasion" in an enactment of "socio-technocratic optimism." Obama's tweet matches this description. He provides an incipient story—specifically, a story about what might happen in the future. This story relies on an ethics that is connected to scientific claims, most significantly the idea that when aggregated with others' actions, one's decisions could have an impact on a nation's mortality rates. Specifically, If people would listen to the epidemiological experts and self-quarantine, a more positive outcome with a "flattened" curve could be achieved.

Another political leader, president Donald Trump, was also vocal about COVID-19. Particularly notorious were his statements about treatments for the virus that the vast majority of the scientific community deemed dubious, at best, or just flat out wrong. For instance, a CNBC

DOI: 10.4324/9781003561019-5

article posted online on May 18, 2020, quotes Trump as saying, "I'm taking it, hydroxychloroquine. Right now, yeah. Couple of weeks ago, I started taking it. Cause I think it's good, I've heard a lot of good stories" (Lovelace Jr. and Breuninger 2020). In response, Dr. Michael Osterholm (director of the Center for Infectious Disease Research and Policy at the University of Minnesota) described the "non-scientific basis on which [Trump's comments] were stated." Dr. Osterholm called the problem "an issue about messaging."[2]

But describing COVID-19 misinformation as an issue about messaging is inaccurate and, in this case, led to ineffective responses to Trump's (and others') statements. This concept of a messaging problem only makes sense within a top-down model of science communication that is prescriptive in nature. Osterholm assumed that scientific information sharing should happen from the top down. That is, scientists do the research; then, they communicate their findings to the public. This is a prescriptive model of how science communication *should* occur, but it is not how scientific ideas actually always circulate across and through social groups. In the top-down model, a problem of messaging indicates a problem of transmitting "the science" to the public. However, the pandemic has made glaringly clear what previous research had already revealed: that this is not the only—nor even the usual—model of the how health knowledge circulates in public discourses (Briggs and Hallin 2016). Across a range of domains in everyday life and professional public/global health contexts, knowledge and opinions about scientific findings often circulate through stories. As Trump stated, he's "heard a lot of good stories"—and non-scientists (lay people) may be active participants in creating and responding to such stories.

If this chapter seems out of place within the context of this book as a whole, it is because it is. The virus forced its way into the book just as it forced its way into people's lives around the world. I was, I thought, wrapping up the Global Health Discourses project when the pandemic began. But the pandemic disrupted my ability to write this book. And as the pandemic progressed, I realized that I was witnessing the development and negotiation of public and global health claims and perspectives. Unfortunately, this became an opportunity to analyze how scientists and the public tried to make sense of a new illness through storytelling in real time.

As with all stories, COVID-19 narratives were not only about the present moment. Rather, they drew on understandings of past events and linked the present to an imagined future—usually a techno-optimistic one in which the pandemic would come to an end. These stories involved what Vincanne Adams, Michelle Murphy, and Adele E. Clarke (2009) call speculative forecast, a kind of "predictable uncertainty" that "leads to anticipation as an *affective state*" (247, emphasis in original). As discussed in Chapter 3, in global health stories the affective state of anticipation most commonly invoked was that of liable affect, which racialized conditions of vulnerability. Public health stories in the United States about the pandemic, on the other hand, leaned heavily on empowering affect. As I will show in this chapter, the emplotment of empowering affect in techno-optimistic stories about COVID-19 foreclosed the possibility of alternative futures in which socioeconomic inequities disproportionately impacting BIPOC (Black, Indigenous, and People of Color) Americans might have been addressed.

While COVID-19 stories were also about ethics and economics (the subjects of Chapters 3 and 4), what I noticed most in the context of my ongoing research project was how epistemic values were emplotted. As I will show, techno-optimistic plots shaped public discourses from the beginning of the pandemic onward: in the uptake of the concept of flattening the curve, debates about sending children back to school, the promotion of the unproven treatment ivermectin, and, finally, the development of COVID-19 vaccines using mRNA technology. In this chapter, I will also ask: what sorts of alternative imagined futures—and thus alternative actions—did techno-optimistic stories preclude? And why did the rare narratives that advocated for structural change instead of efforts that would facilitate a "return to normal" fail to gain traction?

Key Concepts: Emplotment and Epistemic Values

Emplotment is the semiotic process through which plots are created. It refers to the ways that the building blocks of stories are arranged into a coherent whole, linking "agents, goals, means, circumstances, [and] unexpected results" (Ricoeur 1984: 53, 65–66). Often, stories link events that are not temporally contiguous (i.e., they do not occur one right after another in real time). This leads storytelling audiences and analysts alike to think about the question, "Why do narrators select these… events to temporally juxtapose and not others?" (Ochs 2004: 270–271). Placing events together in a story—events that may have happened hours, days, months, or years apart—provides an implicit analysis that suggests that one event caused or influenced the other.

Emplotment also often relates time to place, and often, connects multiple spaces or places (Baynham 2015; Bakhtin 1981). Stories can evoke culturally significant senses of place by drawing upon the social history and already established values associated with specific places as a kind of shorthand in the process of making meaning together (Basso 1988). Of particular significance for my analysis of global health emplotment is how the many disparate sites and spaces of global health may become understood as linked to one another, as well as how health interventions come to be known as spatially generalized (in other words, able to be applied to any population globally). But my examination of techno-optimistic emplotment in this chapter shows that the key element for understanding the epistemic values of global health stories is time, especially imaginative projections of what the future may hold.

Emplotment plays a key part in the constitution of relations between relations—in other words, the constitution of values. In this chapter I focus on *epistemic values*. The study of epistemic values concerns itself with how people define and distinguish knowledge, especially why people value knowledge in comparison with other epistemic claims such as "true belief" (Pritchard 2007). For scientists, the difference between these two is that knowledge, unlike other claims, is arrived at through reliable and repeatable methods. Think of the adage that "a broken clock is right twice a day." This pithy phrase suggests that merely being correct in two instances without a reliable method for arriving at one's "true belief" is not as valuable as "knowledge" that results from being correct because of a confirmable method for finding answers on multiple occasions. The latter, it should be noted, is privileged in part because it provides the ability to make predictions about the future.

In scientific medicine and public/global health, being knowledgeable is often associated with the term expertise. Expertise is itself "implicated in semistable hierarchies of value that authorize particular ways of seeing and speaking as expert" (Carr 2010: 18). Significantly, scientists gain some of their authority as knowledge producers through their insistence that their methodologies are divorced from creative communicative processes (Ochs, Gonzales, and Jacoby 1996: 329–330). However, storytelling and other creative communicative actions are a key part of the everyday activities that produce scientific knowledge (Wolfgram 2016: 34; Ochs, Gonzales, and Jacoby 1996). The stories that global health professionals tell in public discourses (e.g., opinion pieces, appearances on news shows, YouTube videos, websites) showcase expertise and link this expertise to values of the specialized subculture of medicine. This includes reliance on quantitative data and the use of laboratories (e.g., chemical analysis) for the purposes of diagnosis, because these activities are understood to be more accurate for knowledge production than other methods. In terms of the definition of value I utilize in this book, these epistemic values establish relationships between illnesses and population-level interventions in terms of relationships between methodologies and claims of truth.

The Building Blocks of Techno-Optimism

As part of my broader project to understand global health discourses (before and beyond the COVID-19 pandemic), in August of 2020

I watched and analyzed the ten most viewed videos on the YouTube channels of three Atlanta-area non-profit organizations (NPOs): the CDC Foundation, CHAMPS Health, and the Task Force for Global Health. Twenty of these thirty videos contained elements of techno-optimism. In these twenty videos, I identified five plot elements—what I call the building blocks of techno-optimism—that were repeated over and over (see also Black 2021). All five of these building blocks could be found in almost every one of the twenty videos that I watched:

1 A statement of a biomedicalized problem (introducing the villain): there are many different ways that an illness may be conceptualized—for instance, as a moral failing of the individual, or as a symptom of the failure of the government, the community, or the dominant economic system. Biomedicalization entails narrowing the scope of cause and effect to human bodies and pathogens. Illness is presented as an individual problem, rather than a social, institutional, political, or economic one. Such individual problems can then be conceptualized as able to be overcome through a complex array of scientific medical institutions and interventions (Clarke et al. 2003; Moyer and Nguyen 2016).
2 A discussion of actions that a global health professional or organization has taken, is taking, or will be taking (setting the stage): this plot element provides background information that contextualizes a technological intervention. Often, it entails a series of actions related to or in preparation for a technological fix.
3 An emphasis on technology as a fix (a hero emerges): a usually novel technological development (e.g., a new medicine or treatment) is presented as the hero of the story that is prepared to confront the biomedicalized problem.
4 Spatial and/or epidemiological generalization: the technological fix is suggested to be applicable more broadly—either to other locations around the world or to other biomedicalized problems.
5 Projection to a hopeful future: a vision of the future is provided, often in which the technological development has solved the biomedicalized problem.

These plot elements are central to the (re)production of global health's epistemic values. They encourage biomedicalization of health issues in part because if bodies are self-contained units, then it is possible to identify with scientific precision when something changes about a body or a pathogen enters a body. The causal links between things like poverty and illness are less direct and not amenable to experimental or laboratory study, though statistical analysis does provide some indication of the connections between the two.

In terms of the theorization of value I utilize in this book, these building blocks of techno-optimistic stories (re)create a relationship between health practitioners and target populations for interventions, mediated by a relationship between a biomedicalized problem and a technological (often, pharmaceutical) solution. This solution is then projected into an imagined future in which the biomedicalized problem has been overcome. In this chapter, my analysis of public discourses in the emerging COVID-19 pandemic showcases how these five plot elements were deployed in both scientific narratives and pseudo-scientific misinformation to reproduce the epistemic values of public and global health.

"Flattening the Curve" as a Techno-Optimistic Story

Barack Obama's tweet about flattening the curve repeated details and explanations that have been traced back to an article titled "Flattening the Curve," published on February 29, 2020, in *The Economist*, which included a similar graph (image not included due to copyright issues). This graph was itself adapted from a 2007 CDC publication on how to prepare for an influenza epidemic (see Figure 5.1) (CDC 2007).[3] The graph and the title of *The Economist* article quickly circulated through social media posts and into the speeches of politicians and public health experts

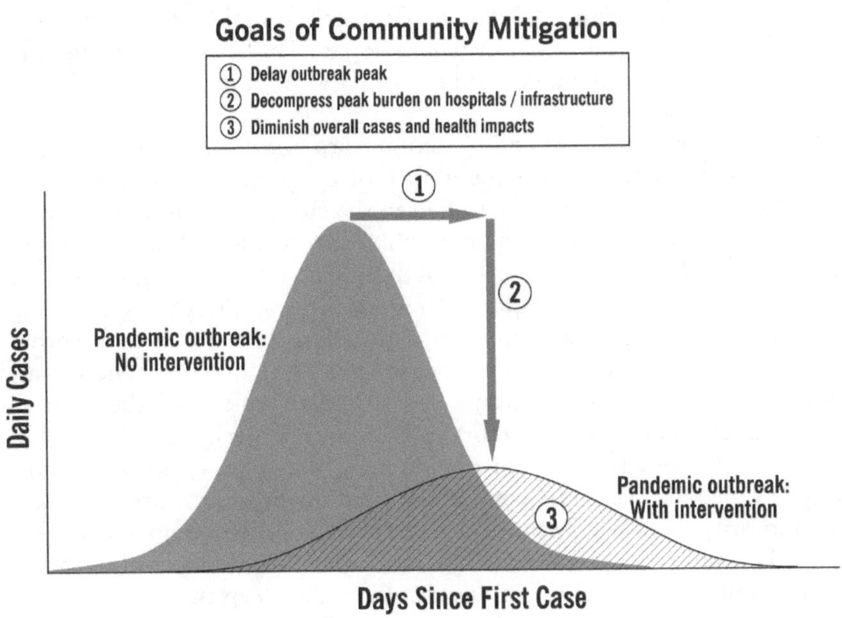

Figure 5.1 CDC Flatten the Curve Graphic (CDC 2007: 18).

around the world, especially after Dr. Drew Harris tweeted a revised version with a horizontal line labeled "healthcare system capacity" just above the flattened curve and slicing through the un-flattened curve (image not included due to copyright issues).[4] Soon after, flattening the curve had gone viral (including in Obama's tweet), circulating in millions of users' social media posts. By November of 2020, the hashtag *#FlattenTheCurve* had been used over 1.5 million times on Instagram (Li and Molder 2021: 899).

Unlike these graphic recontextualizations, the source image—a CDC graph from long before the pandemic—had also included a list of three goals: delay the peak of the outbreak, lessen the burden on hospitals and infrastructure, and diminish the overall number of cases and impact on health (Figure 5.1). In the 2007 CDC publication, the concept of flattening the curve centered around the use of "early, targeted, layered use of non-pharmaceutical interventions" to decrease the peak number of infected individuals and also reduce the total number of cases in the long term, in order to "buy time" for the creation of a vaccine (CDC 2007: 9). Even in its inception, then, flattening the curve was not just optimistic—it was techno-optimistic, focusing on ameliorating conditions until a novel technological intervention could end an epidemic.

During the COVID-19 pandemic, the phrase "buying time" was repeated, sometimes word for word. For instance, a 2020 University of Michigan health blog explains, "[flattening the curve] buys us time for university and government scientists, and industry, to create new therapies, medications and potentially a vaccine" (Gavin 2020).[5] Actions in the present are linked to the future development of new technologies. This idea of "buying time" emplots a future-oriented, hopeful outlook linked to the creation of a new medical technology.

However, this simplistic call to action does not examine the impact of socioeconomic difference on the ability of different groups of people to complete the actions necessary to flatten the curve—for instance, to work from home, pay for high-speed internet in order to allow children to attend school remotely. In addition, many of those who became categorized as essential workers and were required to work in-person were also low-wage workers. How might pandemic responses have progressed differently if narratives and calls to action had focused less on technological heroes and more on interventions that addressed socioeconomics and the need for structural changes (discussed more later in the chapter)?

In and of itself, the concept of flattening the curve is not technologically oriented. It does invite viewers to orient toward the future: "Invoking the authority of (albeit hypothetical) data, it seeks to orient its audience towards a collectively imagined future where the slowly rolling hill of manageable COVID-19 infections displaces the steep mountain of cases that quickly overwhelms healthcare capacity" (Storz and Wynfield 2020). During 2020, the graphic and the phrase "flatten the curve" provided an incipient optimistic narrative—alongside the pessimistic alternative of what would happen without action—to be filled in with content as it circulated and was recontextualized online and offline.

A CDC Webinar Story

Not surprisingly (given its origins), "flatten the curve" also circulated in CDC discourses during the pandemic. One example of this occurred on March 30, 2020, when much of the United States was first entering into a period of extended lockdown. On that date, Dr. Jay C. Butler led a CDC webinar titled "Update for Private Sector Organizations on the 2019 Coronavirus Disease (COVID-19) Response."[6] This would become one of 100 videos on YouTube tagged by CDC as *#COVID-19 Webinar and Partner Calls*. Before becoming the Deputy Director for Infectious Diseases at CDC, Dr. Butler served for over twenty-two years in the Commissioned Corps of the US Public Health Service and directed CDC's 2009 H1N1 Pandemic Vaccine Task Force.[7] Though the 2007 CDC publication that features the flatten the curve graphic has no listed authors, it is possible that Butler participated in the creation of that publication. The 2020 COVID-19 webinar took the form of Butler responding to questions previously submitted by CDC "partners." I emailed the webinar host, Dr. Janelle Peralez Gunn,[8] to ask who these partners were that had submitted questions. She responded that they had many questions from different types of entities, but she remembered mostly NPOs and private companies participating.

At the beginning of the recorded webinar, after a brief introduction by Peralez Gunn, Butler begins with an introduction of his own:

Excerpt 14: CDC Story Part 1 (starting at 1 min 14 sec)

> Good afternoon everybody, good morning to those of you out on the west coast. Ahm, today's March thirtieth. So it's interesting to think, it was December thirty-first that the world was first notified of the cluster of pneumonia cases that occurred in Wuhan China. Ah so just a reflection before we get started, is we are here to talk about a pandemic caused by a virus and a disease that we didn't know existed only three months ago. And it just—it's both humbling and fairly stunning to think how much the world can change in only three months. Of course, as of today, the virus has spread pretty much around the world, there's been laboratory confirmed cases in over two hundred countries now; there's almost certainly some bias in that depending on where testing capacity is, but the virus has now been documented for several weeks on all the inhabited continents of the earth.

These introductory comments—a "reflection before we get started"—are the beginning of a story about the virus and public health responses to it.

This story takes shape as Butler connects the past to the present. He uses the temporal deictic "today" and the date, March 30th, then links this present moment with a past moment—December 31st—when Wuhan China first notified the world about a cluster of pneumonia cases (lines 02–04). Returning to the present, Butler notes that the day on which he is speaking is a three-month anniversary (line 06), and he describes the intervening months as a time of "stunning" change (line 07).

Here, Butler is also beginning to emplot techno-optimism using some of the five building blocks of techno-optimistic global health storytelling. Though some connections remain implicit, COVID-19 is framed as a biomedicalized problem. This is especially evident in the description of "laboratory confirmed cases" and "testing capacity," whereby the medicalized illness is linked to laboratories and a medical technology (lines 09 and 11). In doing so, Butler indexes epistemic concepts common in the medical sciences, namely, reliance on data and the use of chemical analysis in diagnosis. Butler also generalizes spatially, explaining that COVID-19 has now been found on all inhabited continents on earth (line 12).

Butler continues his presentation. Over the next four minutes, he overviews some facts that many people now take for granted but that were just being discovered at the time of the webinar. For instance, he notes that the United States has the most laboratory-confirmed cases of any country, that older people and those with underlying health conditions are at highest risk of severe illness, that the vast majority of people who are infected will recover; and that even asymptomatic infected individuals may have high viral loads and transmit the virus.

After this, Butler shifts to a discussion of how to mitigate transmission of the virus. This is when he introduces the concept of flattening the curve:

Excerpt 15: CDC Story Part 2 (starting at 6 min 16 sec)

01 I think everyone is aware of the goal of flattening the curve? That's become a
02 household term now. The overall goal there is to distribute the impact of the
03 pandemic over as long a period as possible in order to maintain critical
04 infrastructure, and particularly to keep the health care system from becoming
05 overwhelmed.

Here, flattening the curve is not overtly techno-optimistic. In recognition of its wide circulation in public discourses, Butler describes flatten the curve as a household term, and then notes that the goal of flattening the curve is to keep the healthcare system from becoming overwhelmed. Next, he spends about two minutes describing interventions that do not involve novel technologies, such as masking (mentioned at this early point in the pandemic as a potential tool for mitigation), school closures, and social distancing.

After this, though, Butler shifts toward a techno-optimistic perspective as he bookends his discussion of mitigation efforts by returning to flattening the curve:

Excerpt 16: CDC Story Part 3 (starting at 8 min 22 sec)

01 These community mitigation measures are… an important part of what we do
02 to flatten the curve until we know more about the status of any chemo-
03 prophylactic agents—right now there are basically none, there are therapeutic
04 agents that are under study. And we certainly can talk more about that if you
05 would like. A vaccine is probably at best twelve to eighteen months down the
06 road before that would be available for more widespread use.

Recall that Butler had connected the present moment to a past start date for the pandemic at the beginning of his talk. Here, Butler reaches forward in time to link the present to an imagined future. He uses the temporal preposition "until," the temporal deictic "right now," and the subjunctive mood "would be" to provide a sense that in the current moment, people are waiting for an effective novel technological intervention to be developed (lines 02, 03, and 06). In an imagined future, "chemo-prophylactic agents" (in other words, pharmaceuticals) are positioned as a hero who may or may not be able to defeat—or at least slow—the villain (COVID-19) in the near or medium term (lines 02–03). Meanwhile, the whole world waits for another hero—a vaccine (line 05).

Over the course of eight minutes, Dr. Butler links the present moment (late March 2020) to a past event (a cluster of pneumonia cases) in order to delineate the start of the pandemic, while also linking that present to an imagined future that would mark the end of the pandemic with the development of a vaccine. In this case, flattening the curve is an action that is being taken/will be taken, setting the stage for a vaccine hero to emerge. Tense markers, temporal deictics, and temporal prepositions, along with the grammatical organization of phrases and sentences in juxtaposition with one another, emplot this as a techno-optimistic story for an immediate audience (primarily NPOs and private companies) and for imagined future audiences for the recording.

Complementary Futures and Antiheroes

This framing of COVID-19 as a biomedicalized problem awaiting a technological hero is not wrong. In fact, as my discussions with scientific experts demonstrate (see below), vaccines are indeed a key viable long-term scientific solution that saved many lives during the pandemic. Furthermore, the quick development of effective vaccines against COVID-19 using novel mRNA technology was a remarkable achievement. At the same time, this version of the story is incomplete. Other complementary solutions—including some that were an integral part of flattening the curve—were simply not considered to be part of viable long-term resolutions. These potential solutions included actions such as making changes to crowded meat-packing facility design, installing better HVAC and ventilation in crowded buildings, and creating smaller classes at schools. But these options required money and changes to existing institutions and regulations; and for some political actors, these were not thought to be acceptable because they involved government oversight of private companies.

These were potential actions that would have required changes to the economic and political status quo, something that global and public health have long resisted (Biehl 2007). This and other concerns, alongside the significant income to be made selling vaccines and medicines, pushed public and global health to high-value pharmaceutical interventions and other technological interventions during the COVID-19 pandemic. But what of the alternatives? What about interventions that might have played the role of antiheroes (central characters that lack conventional heroic qualities and attributes) within the narrative strictures of neoliberal capitalism?

These antiheroes did make their way into public discourses at times but had little uptake. The antihero stories just did not circulate as widely or as quickly as their alternatives. Here I examine how this process played out locally, in the home communities of public health professionals themselves, in Decatur, Georgia. In December 2020, Decaturish (a local Decatur, Georgia online news site) published a letter to the editor that addressed the question of reopening public schools. The school closing that some of us thought would last two or three weeks at most in March 2020 had dragged on through the end of that school year and halfway into the next. And while most Decatur parents were strong proponents of science-based school policies designed to protect the health of children and other community members, many were also extremely tired and anxious about the impact that so much time out of school was having on children's mental health and scholarly progress.

The letter to the editor was titled "Dear Decaturish—City Schools of Decatur Should Offer In-Person Learning Option for All Students." This piece was penned by eighteen public and global health professionals who were also parents of students in the Decatur school district (Brooks et al. 2020).[9] One of the co-authors was Nancy Messonnier, who signed as a private citizen but who was in charge of CDC's COVID-19 taskforce at that time (and was regularly in the national news). At around the same time that the letter was published, some homes in my neighborhood also sprouted yellow lawn signs that featured a message printed in black: "our children deserve better, SAFE CHOICE NOW" (referring to the idea that parents should have the choice to safely send their kids back to school).

Soon afterward, an Associated Press article about what was happening in "CDC's Backyard" described strain in the community about the return to school, explaining, "Around Decatur, neighbors dodged the issue in polite conversation as tensions rose during school board meetings and on social media" (Press 2021).[10] Based on my own experience, I would say that it was not that neighbors dodged the issue, precisely, but rather that many were careful about how they raised the question of a return to school. After all, it was not as if a significant number of people in our area were denying the significance of COVID-19 (e.g., arguing that it was just like the flu or that it was made up by the government). In other words, most residents were approaching the question of school reopening with the same basic set of epistemic values that were rooted in science and medicine. The distinctions in opinion were more subtle, taking the form of a disagreement about what "the science" suggested was the best course of action.

This subtlety is reflected in the first sentence of the Decaturish letter to the editor, which explains that the authors' purpose is to express "concerns about the narrow use and misrepresentation of science" in City Schools of Decatur's policy decision regarding older students and in-person learning. The school district had just determined that sixth to twelfth graders would not have the option of a return to in-person learning, because they felt that it was unfeasible to reduce class sizes for the older students. Meanwhile, younger children were allowed the option to return, because they were already in smaller classes that enabled students to be spaced further apart and have less contact with one another. The editorial argues that school administrators who made this decision were misreading available scientific evidence and that they were focusing narrowly on COVID-19 infections when they ought to have also been thinking more broadly about students' physical and mental health.

The editorial continues, "Research conducted throughout Europe, Asia and Australia has shown very little transmission in schools, with a wide variety of mitigation measures in place." Here, the present perfect tense ("has shown") indicates an already completed action: research already conducted. In terms of emplotment, this declaration serves a similar role to the "what has been done/what is being done" building block of techno-optimistic stories, creating relevant story setting.

In a third paragraph, the authors provide a partial list of CDC's mitigation strategies. This includes "the use of face coverings, physical distancing, environmental hygiene, and cohorting." The repetition of the term "mitigation" in this paragraph serves as a rhetorical link between what CDC recommends and what was mentioned earlier—namely, previous research on appropriate actions to reduce transmission in other parts of the world. The authors then argue that it is possible to achieve similarly low levels of transmission through a "variety of approaches (e.g., hybrid models that split the school population for alternating days)." This contrasts with the City Schools of Decatur's decision that class cohorts were to be required to be smaller than fifteen students.

This letter to the editor does not present a techno-optimistic story. Instead, it presents a pessimistic view of a potentially negative future facilitated by the school district's restriction of older children from in-person education. The authors cite a "great deal of evidence that long term virtual instruction is damaging many students' learning and development and exacerbates already existing inequities in educational outcomes"; they mention that "early indications show the very negative impact of virtual learning on academic achievement"; and they state, "There is extensive evidence that connection to schools and important adults in school protects youth from a host of risks including poor mental health and substance abuse."

The way to avoid this negative imagined future, the authors suggest, is to allow older children to go back to in-person learning with mitigation measures in place. In the CDC story about flattening the curve, vaccines played the role of the hero. Here, vaccines do not appear as part of the discussion, nor is the story truly techno-optimistic in nature. Still, there is a similarity between this and the flatten-the-curve story: a lack of action will lead to something bad happening. Both are also rooted in a conviction that science provides the answers to questions about what actions should be taken.

How might this same story have been told in a more compelling way? Much of the letter is phrased in the negative: it describes why the actions of City Schools of Decatur officials were incorrect. On the other hand, the authors do mention mitigation strategies. This provides a potential cast of antihero characters that together might be presented as fending off COVID-19. Learning from techno-optimistic storytelling, I would suggest that stories featuring these sorts of antiheroes would do well to provide an alternative story trajectory that focuses on a future in which the antagonist (in this case, the virus) has been overcome, or at least kept at bay. The editorial was steeped in scientific writing principles such as the need to disprove previous approaches. But such principles do not transfer easily or effectively from the realm of scholarly white papers to the world of public discourses.

Still, whether through the letter to the editor or other channels, the message was clearly received, probably in part due to the institutional authority associated with the authors. Less than a month later, middle school and high school officials were at work on an in-person learning timeline and implementation plan. It helped that early vaccines were also starting to become available to teachers. By early March of 2021, middle school and high school students were back to in-person learning. Then, in early October of 2021, the school district established a Public Health, Medical, and Science COVID-19 Advisory team. The team included Dr. Messonnier (who had resigned from CDC in May of 2021). Of the team's eleven members, six were current CDC employees and all had considerable experience in public health.[11]

Most school districts were not able to rely on such high-level public health expertise among their parents, and in any case not all communities foregrounded the epistemic values of science to shape their COVID-19 policies. For the purposes of this chapter, one significant facet of the Decaturish editorial is that it showcases the variability that can be found within the confines of the epistemic values of public and global health. In addition, interventions need not be technologically oriented to be optimistic in nature. Outside of the Decatur/CDC bubble, one thing that might help to push conversations in new directions would be to develop some non-techno-optimistic global and public health stories that more effectively leverage the emplotment of antiheroes, especially in stories that advocate for structural change. Public and global health already have a range of these antiheroes at their disposal. For instance, improving ventilation in schools and factories would help mitigate not only COVID-19 but a host of other health issues. Implementation of sick-leave policies would greatly impact a number of inequities in health, education, and beyond. The creation of persuasive, future-oriented stories centered around these alternative protagonists might help to shift conversations away from antagonistic and seemingly intractable arguments. Such an emphasis on equity and structural changes also aligns with efforts to decolonize public and global health by shifting interventions away from those that reproduce or reinforce the socioeconomic status quo.

Hydroxychloroquine, Ivermectin, and Other Techno-Optimistic Misinformation

While it might seem that COVID-19 pseudo-therapies promoted by Donald Trump and others were also antiheroes, in reality they fit the mold of techno-optimistic heroes. In 2020 and beyond, one of the most intractable political-health arguments involved pseudo-scientific treatments for the virus such as hydroxychloroquine and ivermectin. The latter two were promoted by anti-vaxxers and some on the far right of the political spectrum (who may or may not have been anti-vaccine). Misinformation about drugs such as hydroxychloroquine and ivermectin is clearly not equivalent to well-founded scientific information about concepts like flattening the curve and proven treatments such as vaccines. Still, in contrast to the commonly articulated idea that support for these alternative treatments was anti-science, in this section I argue that these stories share something in common with stories about vaccines: an underlying techno-optimism (see also Berlivet and Löwy 2020).

Actually, accurate stories about vaccine efficacy and inaccurate stories about alternative drug treatments shared *two* things in common: techno-optimism and a connection to profitable markets. At one point, two large groups of physicians pushing ivermectin had been charging hundreds or even a thousand dollars to get an online appointment for a prescription for the drug (Goldhill 2022).[12] While the alternative-treatments trend was surely financially motivated, it was also more than that. These stories offered counter-narratives rooted in distrust of government, the scientific establishment, and intellectualism in general (Goldhill 2022)—but counter-narratives that were nonetheless techno-optimistic in nature.

Anthropological analysis of the rise of hydroxychloroquine and ivermectin treatments has led scholars to re-examine the question of "Who is entitled to participate in the shaping and validation of new medical knowledge and practices?" (Berlivet and Löwy 2020: 527). Past inequities in public and global health research attest to the importance of this question. For instance, during the early years of the HIV pandemic in the United States, activists pushed back against ethical rules for the organization of clinical trials in order to accelerate the development of treatment at a time when many were dying. Dr. Anthony Fauci, who would become central in debates about science, medicine, and COVID-19, notably played a key role in these negotiations about HIV treatment (Berlivet and Löwy 2020: 531–532, 536).

During the COVID-19 pandemic, however, valid critical viewpoints on scientific knowledge production were hijacked by rhetorically gifted salespeople who made a profit off of the supposed miracle tonics of hydroxychloroquine and ivermectin. This was made possible through these critics' alliances with charismatic political/media figures who mobilized populist support by rejecting scientific "elites." The critique of so-called elites (ironically, critiques often made by elite politicians and pundits) cast suspicion on epidemiologists while telling people to trust physicians (Berlivet and Löwy 2020). In the recording discussed below, for instance, Senator Ron Johnson described physicians by saying, "these are the medical practitioners, the *heroes*, that experts in the ivory towers and media have chosen to ignore and vilify." Doctors undergo years of schooling and training that rival or exceed that of epidemiologists, and many public health professionals also have medical degrees. Still, this idea of physicians doing "real" work in contrast to epidemiology seemed to resonate with conservative discourses that already had working-class and business-oriented pretensions. Another reason this tack may have been effective is that many people did not know much about epidemiologists or epidemiology, while they had been receiving medical care from physicians for their whole lives. In addition, everybody loves a good underdog story.

A Homeland Security Story

Despite their lack of basis in scientific fact, narratives about alternative treatments-as-pseudo-heroes emplotted many of the same epistemic values that are mobilized in other public and global health stories. One example of this emplotment comes from a US Senate Homeland Security Committee meeting. This meeting, with a Focus on Early Treatment of COVID-19, occurred on December 8, 2020 (around the time of the publication of the Decaturish letter to the editor). Republican senator Ron Johnson had invited Dr. Pierre Kory and a number of other medical professionals to testify at this meeting. He extended this invitation after advisers to then-President Trump pressured Johnson to start a campaign to get the Food and Drug Administration (FDA) to reauthorize the use of hydroxychloroquine as a treatment for COVID-19. Despite the lack of a clear connection to the mandate of the US Senate Committee on Homeland Security and Governmental Affairs, the senator leveraged his position as chairman of the committee to host public meetings with notable doctors who were promoting the drug.[13]

Dr. Kory—who was one of the headliners of these meetings—was the leader of a newly created NPO, the Front-Line COVID-19 Critical Care Alliance (note how this mirrors the myriad other NPOs associated with global health). According to an in-depth investigation in 2022 about long COVID patients (patients experiencing long-lasting health problems following infection with COVID-19) and ivermectin, Dr. Kory "began touting ivermectin out of desperation to combat the virus, but he has increasingly embraced vaccine skepticism and rejected Big Pharma and conventional medicine. He has found a large online audience" (Goldhill 2022).[14] Indeed, Kory appeared on Fox News and the Joe Rogan podcast and was promoted by a secretive Christian policy organization called the Council for National Policy (Goldhill 2022).

The December 2020 Homeland Security hearing, which was recorded and posted on YouTube (like the other videos analyzed in this chapter), begins with introductory comments by Senator Johnson. In his introduction, Johnson references a previous hearing that he says is complementary to this second hearing. The previous hearing had featured testimony by Dr. Peter McCullouch, who was an anti-COVID-vaccine doctor who produced a popular podcast with the far-right "America Out Loud Network." After appearing at these Homeland Security meetings, McCullouch was fired from his position at Baylor University Medical center for spreading misinformation about COVID-19, treatments, and vaccines.[15]

In the second Homeland Security meeting recording—the one featuring Dr. Kory—Senator Johnson begins with two slides from the previous presentation.[16] The first slide is a visual of what McCullouch had discussed as "four pillars of pandemic response." As the slide is displayed, Johnson explains,

Excerpt 17: Homeland Security Story Part 1 (starting at 44 sec)

> Sen. Johnson: The first pillar is contagion control. And of course we've done that with (waves hands) social distancing, and economic shutdowns, masks, all those types of things. The second pillar is early home treatment. The third is late-stage hospital treatment, and the fourth is vaccination.

Next, Johnson asks for a second slide from the previous meeting to be displayed. This slide features medical terms superimposed on a graph representing the stages of severe COVID and untreated mortality risk from day 0 symptom onset to thirty days. The slide also includes a citation to the Baylor University Medical Center Proceedings, which is in fact a peer-reviewed journal. Johnson explains that the second slide visualizes the "three stages of COVID"—viral replication, cytokine storm, and microthrombosis—which was an accurate description of available scientific medical understandings of how the virus infects human hosts. As with the flatten-the-curve concept, this use of charts and graphs is part of an aesthetics of scientific discourse that invokes biomedical authority.

Johnson then states (1 min 21 sec), "the goal of this hearing is identical to the goal of our first hearing: to discuss early treatment options that attack the disease in the first stage by limiting viral replication." He also explains (1 min 43 sec), "This is how Tamiflu works in limiting the severity of the flu. It is how we approach every other disease. Early detection allows for early treatment, and better outcomes. Seems like a pretty commonsense approach to me." Rather than a critique of science, Johnson emphasizes how the intervention that he is advocating is similar to other science-based interventions.

All the plot elements of a techno-optimistic narrative appear in Senator Johnson's introduction: a statement of a biomedicalized problem (the three stages of COVID); an indication of what has been done or is being done ("we've done that with social distancing, and economic shutdowns, masks"); technology as a solution (the hearing will discuss early treatment options—meaning hydroxychloroquine and ivermectin); biomedical and/or spatial generalization ("It's how we approach every other disease"); and projection to a hopeful future ("Early detection allows for early treatment, and better outcomes").

After Johnson's introduction, two physicians provide testimony to argue that scientific inquiry is being stifled by big government and pharmaceutical intervention. Then Dr. Kory begins his speech. Excerpt 18 is taken from a published written version of Kory's comments that was circulated prior to the Homeland Security meeting. In his live speech, Kory diverged significantly from these written remarks in ways that were difficult to follow, though the same major plot elements and points can be found.

Excerpt 18: Homeland Security Story Part 2 (Dr. Kory)

01 Although we, like many, are extremely encouraged by the apparent successes
02 in developing effective vaccines, we also are dismayed at the near complete
03 absence of guidance and research on effective early, at-home, or preventative
04 treatment options apart from vaccines, a reality we find unconscionable. Our
05 hospitals are overflowing with over 100,000 COVID-19 patients admitted,
06 and new record deaths are reported each passing day. It will take months for
07 the vaccine to be distributed to the general public and further time to have
08 sufficient impact in this crisis, so we are here to stress the need for effective
09 early treatment. My organization of critical care specialists have spent the
10 almost nine months tirelessly reviewing the scientific literature to gain insight
11 into this virus and the disease process and to develop effective treatment
12 protocols… And so, it is with great pride as well as significant optimism, that
13 I am here to report that our group, led by Professor Paul E. Marik, has
14 developed a highly effective protocol for preventing and early treatment of
15 COVID-19. In the last 3–4 months, emerging publications provide conclusive
16 data on the profound efficacy of the anti-parasite, anti-viral drug, anti-
17 inflammatory agent called ivermectin in all stages of the disease.

Like Senator Johnson's introduction, this statement includes four of the five plot elements of techno-optimistic global health stories. It also uses "effective" five times (lines 02, 03, 08, 11, and 14). Dr. Kory identifies a biomedicalized problem, stating that there is an absence of research on early treatments and hospitals overflowing (lines 02–05); he explains what has been done/what is being done ("My organization of critical care specialists have…" lines 09–12); he indicates that technology is the answer—in this case, ivermectin (lines 16–17); and he projects temporally to a hopeful future ("significant optimism," line 12). Here, the spatial/epidemiological generalization—that this treatment will work on all people in all places—remains unstated but is a central feature of contemporary medical perspectives.

These individuals are not presenting themselves as anti-science. Rather, they are mobilizing key scientific values, such as biomedicalized claims and reliance on evidence and data (what Kory called "emerging publications," lines 15–16), to craft their stories about alternative treatments. Their story is a recontextualization and a (some might say deliberate) re-definition of lexical and narrative features of techno-optimistic global health storytelling. In their critique of the big pharmaceutical powers that be, these doctors nonetheless optimistically imagine a future in which a novel use of existing prophylactic technology will solve the complex problem of the COVID-19 pandemic.

Watching the video of this hearing, it is striking to see how Johnson, Kory, and others seem genuinely committed to the notion that they are fighting against the powers that be to try to save lives. Earlier, the ranking Democratic member of this Senate committee, Senator Peters, had said that the proceedings of the day were political rather than scientific. In response, Dr. Kory replies, "I was discredited as a politician. I am a physician and a man of science" (29 min 11 sec). Without further evidence, it is not possible to determine the degree to which these speakers believe the claims that they are making. However, they are insistent that they are indeed scientists who are interpreting scientific data, despite the fact that the vast majority of scientists disagree with their interpretation; and they are making their arguments through the emplotment of techno-optimistic narratives.

Vaccine Stories: A Techno-Optimistic Future Fulfilled

> I mean this is the problem. Once you realize that it's not going to go away, once you realize that this virus is going to be with us forever, you're just delaying the inevitable. And we're seeing this now in Hong Kong, for example, where they had this zero-tolerance policy and they kept things clamped down, and now it's just spreading everywhere, now they've got the highest rate of transmission in the world. You can only buy time, and the only thing that it makes sense to buy time for is a vaccine.
>
> – James (a global health professional who worked with a governmental organization for many years, then at an NPO, and worked extensively on COVID-19 responses, interview on 03-15-2022, 19 min 24 sec)

> I think it was a success from the vaccine perspective. We didn't get everything we wanted from the vaccine in terms of being able to stop mild infections, but as far as keeping people out of the hospital and preventing deaths, I mean, it was a huge success, and it was fast, it helped prove a new vaccine technology—the mRNA vaccine—which they're now potentially trying to use for a new HIV vaccine.
>
> – Robert (a global health professional who has worked with a governmental organization for many years, interview on 05-13-2022, 18 min 20 sec)

By March 2021 the vaccines that CDC leaders had asked the public to "buy time for" by flattening the curve had arrived. Though pharmaceutical companies created and sold these vaccines, the US government also invested billions—some estimate about twenty billion dollars—in direct spending on the development and manufacturing of the vaccines (Frank, Dach, and Lurie 2021). By and large, global health professionals felt that the development of COVID vaccines were a "huge success," as the above quotes attest. Technologically speaking, this was certainly true, and indicative of the impressive and sometimes unnerving reach and power of scientific medicine and biotechnology in contemporary life.

However, as was the case with infections and deaths during the pandemic, early vaccine distribution and uptake were uneven, and this unevenness was patterned along racialized socioeconomic fault lines. In public discussions about these disparities, commentators tended to mention vaccine "hesitancy" and a distrust of the medical system rooted in a history of medical malpractice and mistreatment, especially among Black Americans (discussed in Chapter 2). But anthropological research on vaccine decision-making concludes that the term "hesitancy" obscures a more complex set of problems that include lack of access to vaccines, structural racism, and "a range of concerns about vaccines that can vary in detail and severity from person to person" (Brunson et al. 2021: 4). It is also likely that low-income individuals lacked trust in medical providers in part because they did not have regular access to health care and were not able to regularly see the same doctors when they did have access, as has been the case in other instances of non-uptake of new medical technologies (e.g., Rapp 1998). There was also great deal of misinformation circulating in public discourses about the safety of the vaccines, as well as some concern and disgruntlement as the public became aware that they would be asked to continue receiving booster shots for the foreseeable future.

With such disparities, concerns, and disgruntlement in mind, when I interviewed global health professionals about vaccines, I was surprised to hear them describe COVID-19 vaccines as a great success story. However, their assessment was fully in line with the commonly held notion that medicine (and science more generally) is a "culture of no culture" (Taylor 2003). That is, "Medical knowledge is understood to be not merely 'cultural' knowledge but *real* knowledge" (Taylor 2003: 556). Doctors and other scientists view such knowledge as based on a qualitatively different type of epistemic claim. The scientific success of vaccine development—utilizing a novel method (mRNA technology) to create a new vaccine that effectively prevented deaths at a speed previously unseen—could be constructed as a success story because that story excised the inequities in access to care and the lack of effective communication about the vaccine. Such muddy details were delimited as being outside the scope of "the science." In this limited sense, public and global health professionals told stories about COVID-19 vaccines that indicated a techno-optimistic future fulfilled.

Leana Wen's Opinion

One public health figure that began touting COVID-19 vaccines soon after their roll-out was Dr. Leana Wen. According to her biography on the George Washington University website, Dr. Wen, who had been Baltimore's Health Commissioner, was "an emergency physician, professor of health policy and management at George Washington University, and a nonresident senior fellow at the Brookings Institution" who also contributed as a columnist for *The Washington Post* and as an analyst on CNN.[17] On April 21, 2021, *The Washington Post* published an editorial by Dr. Wen (2021) titled "The Vaccine Success Story Needs to Be Told." Here is how the editorial begins:

> Recent news coverage is fueling a pernicious narrative: What's the point of getting a covid-19 vaccine if the vaccinated might still get infected, if protection doesn't last that long and if the vaccine itself could lead to dangerous outcomes such as blood clots? Clinicians need to address each concern head-on, and we need the media's help to do it. The science is squarely on our side. Last week, the Centers for Disease Control and Prevention released data on breakthrough coronavirus infections—meaning instances of fully vaccinated people testing positive. The data highlighted how effective vaccination is, but you might not have drawn that conclusion from news reports.

In terms of the five plot elements of techno-optimistic narratives, this introduction presupposes that COVID-19 is being interpreted as a narrowly biomedical problem (rather than, for instance, in part a result of structural inequities or the environmental impacts of unfettered global capitalism forcing humans and animal disease vectors into ever closer and more frequent contact). Here, Dr. Wen is confident that concerns and critiques about the vaccine would be addressed, if only people—getting their information from "news reports" (what she later describes as "the media")—understood "the science" better. As I mentioned at the beginning of this chapter, this is at best an oversimplification about how the majority of Americans obtain and interpret information about COVID-19 and science and medicine in general. Previous scholarship explains that "Biomedical authority models project medical knowledge as embodying hierarchically organized ways of knowing and acting," and biomedical authorities have historically evaluated laypersons (individuals and groups) in terms of their capacity to act in ways that are compatible with these hierarchies (Briggs and Hallin 2016: 205). However, this descriptive (rather than prescriptive) approach to the study of the media circulation of biomedical knowledge indicates that people are active participants in the interpretation and circulation of that knowledge; and also, that the top-down hierarchy of science communication is rooted in a history of racism and colonialism in medicine and public health (Briggs and Hallin 2016).

In her commentary, Wen continues with several statements about the statistics of COVID infections and deaths among vaccinated and unvaccinated individuals. She then suggests, "the media needs to put these numbers into better perspective. No vaccine is 100 percent effective, and the covid-19 vaccines rank high in terms of providing extraordinary protection against infection." This is a summary that falls under the "what we've done" plot element. It is also linked to a spatial generalization in the sense that this vaccine is meant to be universally effective for all people.

After that, Wen's editorial continues with a discussion and clarification of recent data about blood clots in recipients of the Johnson and Johnson vaccine. Finally, she concludes,

> Put simply: More than 567,000 Americans have died from covid-19. Vaccines protect us against this deadly disease and are our pathway back to pre-pandemic life. Science has delivered a remarkable breakthrough, and all of us—from the medical establishment to the government to the media—should be putting the minimal risks into perspective while celebrating the vaccines' overwhelming benefits.

In other words, the techno-optimistic future that scientists had been telling everyone to wait for while they "flattened the curve" is now here. The vaccine is a technological hero, as is "science" ("science has delivered a remarkable breakthrough"). Yet Wen's optimism is still partially unfulfilled, as the imagined future of a return to pre-pandemic life depends on people actually getting the vaccine and future boosters. The problem, in Wen's opinion, is not the science—it is the people. The claims of scientific medicine are sound, based as they are on clear epistemic values about how to produce knowledge.

Wen's argument that humans must change will never be effective, as suggested by the lack of effective scientific medical solutions in response to the perceived intractability of humans-being-humans. What is needed is an approach that incorporates social scientific analysis of local cultural and socioeconomic worlds into the design of public health interventions. For instance, a groundbreaking effort published in July 2021, "Carrying Equity in COVID-19 Vaccination Forward: Guidance Informed by Communities of Color," which included not only public health professionals but also anthropologists, sociologists, and community health workers, makes a number of suggestions for improving vaccination rates (Brunson et al. 2021). Notably, these include structural interventions such as "anchor COVID-19 vaccination for hard hit areas in a holistic recovery process" (27) and "rebuild the public health infrastructure, properly staffing it for community engagement" (31). Simply publishing news stories telling people over and over again that vaccines are safe is not very effective, but providing comprehensive health care which allows people to be in regular contact with doctors and community health workers (establishing real relationships with them) has a proven history of success. These suggestions are not meant to supplant the novel technological intervention of COVID-19 vaccines, but rather to support and expand upon this intervention. However, such an approach would require broadening the epistemic values of public and global health. At the beginning of this chapter, I stated that the epistemic values establish relationships between illnesses and population-level interventions in terms of relationships between methodologies and claims of truth. Incorporating social science into health interventions requires a recalibration of the relationship between methodologies and claims of truth, asking science to more substantively engage with qualitative and ethnographic methodologies (I return to this point in Chapter 7).

Plug and Play Technology

At the beginning of this section, I quoted two global health professionals—James and Robert—who provided positive assessments of COVID-19 vaccines. These quotations are abstracted from interviews I conducted to probe these interviewees' understandings of vaccine development and other health interventions, especially non-techno-optimistic interventions. I spoke with James, a long-time global health official who had worked on COVID-19 responses, about this topic. James was insistent that with an airborne disease such as COVID-19, everyone would eventually become exposed regardless of other interventions. Thus, non-vaccine efforts should be conceptualized as efforts to flatten the curve and reduce burden on the healthcare system while a vaccine was being developed (this is almost word for word what appeared in CDC reports and the CDC webinar).

As our conversation continued, we spoke about the evolution of different COVID-19 variants, and I asked about the role of public health responses in that context:

Excerpt 19: There's No New Science in the Responses (Interview 03-15-2022 starting at 25 min 09 sec)

01 James: I think the responses are pretty straightforward. There's no new
02 science in the responses. I mean, wear a mask, wash your hands, cover your

> cough, I mean do all of those things. Quarantine, isolation, those things have not changed in a hundred years. And I think we have to be prepared to do them… we have to have the credibility, the institutions that are recommending them, so that people actually follow the advice. I think the one big change that we've seen in the last two years is the appearance of all these new platforms for vaccination, the mRNA vaccines and some of these others. I think these are a huge change in our ability to be prepared. You know once we become more comfortable with these vaccines, once we know more about how they behave, how to modify them, and the technology is more widespread for people to produce them, I think that's a huge advantage in the future. Especially if we can transfer that technology to Africa, and some of the places that have really suffered from lack of access.

First, James mentions some of the same public health responses that had been part of the "flattening the curve" discussions early in the pandemic—for instance, in the types of mitigation efforts mentioned in the Decaturish editorial (James also discussed these earlier in our interview). Next, he says that the institutions recommending these actions need to be credible (line 05). In saying this, James is pointing to an earlier moment in our interview when he mentioned how political forces (obliquely referring to Trump and others) had hampered CDC's early response to the pandemic.

After this, James abruptly switches focus to talk about mRNA vaccine technology (lines 07–08). This topic switch should be understood within the larger context of the semi-structured interview in which I was aiming us toward a discussion of non-vaccine interventions. It seems that James wanted to be sure to emphasize the success and significance of the vaccines. His discussion of vaccines remains techno-optimistic even after their development. James uses the temporal conjunction "once" ("once we become more comfortable with these vaccines"), which, when paired with the present tense, indicates an orientation to the future—what can, could, or should happen (lines 09 and 10). The subject and agent of this sentence is "we" (line 10, an unspecified first-person plural that in context seems to refer to the United States as a whole). He envisions becoming more comfortable with the vaccines, understanding more about how they work and how to modify them, and spreading the production technology more widely. In other words, after stating what has been and is being done, James suggests that a next step is spatial generalization of this technological solution to enact a hopeful future. But this future is as yet unfulfilled. "We" need to "transfer that technology to Africa" and other places that have lacked access (lines 13–14).

This is a lofty goal in the current economic configuration of global health—something that James recognizes. He discusses some of the issues involved in such a technological transfer, including health systems strengthening, workforce training, and patent negotiations. Then he returns to the issue of the new mRNA technology that was used to create many of the COVID-19 vaccines:

Excerpt 20: Plug and Play (Interview 03-15-2022 starting at 31 min 15 sec)

> James: I think the mRNA technology is going to be a great boon. It just seems like such a no-hassle platform when you can kind of plug and play, just insert a genome. You can transfer the genetic information that needs to be included in the vaccine by email. ((chuckles)) I mean, you upload a genetic sequence onto one of the gene reservoir sites and anybody can download it and say "oh, that's the sequence I need to prepare to plug into this platform."

This final statement, that "anybody can download it," is especially striking in conjunction with the discussion James and I had just had about issues involved with international transfer of mRNA vaccine technology, in which James made it clear that many countries' health systems did not have the capability to utilize this technology. James knew the challenges involved. While he is speaking in the present tense about the capabilities of this technology, his initial use of the future tense stative verbal construction "going to be" indicates that the present he is speaking about is meant to be positioned within an imagined future. The idea is that "we" have all this great technology, and "now" our task is to make it spatially generalized—and potentially epidemiologically generalized to make vaccines for other diseases—and available to all. Here, a techno-optimistic perspective has the potential to gloss over the structural inequities that make it impossible for the vast majority of humans on the planet to just "download it" or "plug and play" without significant alterations to global economics, institutions, and social structures. This narrative structuring of the epidemiological generalization may in fact discourage attention to such inequities.

Conclusion

Once you see techno-optimism in public and global health you cannot unsee it. This configuration of epistemic values is ever-present in contemporary health discourses in the United States and beyond. In this chapter's examination of emplotment in the narrative constitution of techno-optimism, I have argued that the prevalence and rhetorical power of techno-optimism may limit people's imagining of alternatives (such as advocacy for structural changes). At the same time, the deployment of techno-optimism is expansive—it can be articulated in the service of scientific or pseudo-scientific conclusions alike. Whether truly supported by scientific evidence or not, storytelling plays a key role in continuously reimagining this value system into being.

COVID-19 stories provide an example of the real-time constitution of global health stories. These stories were dominated by plots that utilized the building blocks of techno-optimism. As the previous chapters demonstrated, part of the power of techno-optimism comes from its linking of key epistemic values to prominent ethical and economic values. Global health stories such as those discussed in this chapter presuppose these ethical and economic values in the emplotment of biomedicalization and spatial and epidemiological generalization as well as an imaginative orientation toward the future.

In terms of the COVID-19 pandemic and global health more generally, there are two key takeaways of this discussion. First, scholars, health officials, and pundits should disabuse themselves of the notion that they can easily mitigate health misinformation by labeling it unscientific or anti-science. As examination of Dr. Kory's speech to the US Senate Homeland Security Committee demonstrates, those who voice misinformation may utilize scientific discourses and deploy plot elements of techno-optimism in the service of their claims. At least some of those who adopt stances associated with misinformation do so from what they feel to be a scientific viewpoint. Second, those who hope to advocate for structural changes as a key part of public health interventions need to develop compelling stories that are framed with a positive vision of the future. Perhaps the uptake of storytelling conventions associated with antiheroes could be leveraged to craft an optimism linked to but not wholly rooted in novel technological development.

Notes

1 https://twitter.com/barackobama/status/1238238576141352966?lang=en. Accessed 2/2/2023.
2 https://www.pbs.org/newshour/show/an-infectious-disease-expert-on-the-dangers-of-trumps-non-scientific-claims. Accessed 08/05/2022.
3 https://www.economist.com/briefing/2020/02/29/covid-19-is-now-in-50-countries-and-things-will-get-worse. Accessed 8/11/2022; titled "Flattening the Curve" in the print edition.
4 https://twitter.com/drewaharris/status/1233267475036372992. Accessed 08/16/2022.
5 https://healthblog.uofmhealth.org/wellness-prevention/flattening-curve-for-covid-19-what-does-it-mean-and-how-can-you-help. Accessed 08/11/2022.
6 https://www.youtube.com/watch?v=OdN7NtgV-Bs. Accessed 8/12/2022. Note that there were no visuals used during this webinar other than a title screen.
7 https://www.cdc.gov/about/leadership/leaders/ddid.html. Accessed 08/12/2022.
8 Dr. Peralez Gunn is Associate Director for Policy, Partnerships and Communication for the Division of Nutrition, Physical Activity and Obesity at CDC

9 https://decaturish.com/2020/12/dear-decaturish-city-schools-of-decatur-should-offer-in-person-learning-option-for-all-students/. Accessed 9–13–2022.
10 https://www.wabe.org/in-cdcs-backyard-school-reopening-debate-divides-experts/. Accessed 9/13/2022.
11 https://www.csdecatur.net/Page/4813. Accessed 10/12/22.
12 https://www.statnews.com/2022/07/26/ivermectin-has-become-a-popular-treatment-for-long-covid-with-a-push-from-doctors-with-ties-to-right-wing-political-groups/. Accessed 08/16/2022.
13 https://www.jsonline.com/story/news/politics/2022/08/24/trump-advisors-turned-ron-johnson-push-hydroxychloroquine/7886363001/. Accessed 10/13/22.
14 https://www.statnews.com/2022/07/26/ivermectin-has-become-a-popular-treatment-for-long-covid-with-a-push-from-doctors-with-ties-to-right-wing-political-groups/. Accessed 09/15/2022.
15 https://www.examiner-enterprise.com/story/news/2021/10/06/doctor-fired-baylor-spreading-covid-19-misinformation-finds-supportive-crowd-bartlesville/5995698001/. Accessed 10/13/22.
16 https://www.youtube.com/watch?v=k8RyV3VEDKI. Accessed 10/13/22.
17 https://publichealth.gwu.edu/departments/health-policy-and-management/leana-wen-md-msc_faaem. Accessed 10/18/22.

References

Adams, Vincanne, Michelle Murphy, and Adele E. Clarke. 2009. "Anticipation: Technoscience, Life, Affect, Temporality." *Subjectivity* 28: 246–265.

Bakhtin, Mikhail. 1981. *The Dialogic Imagination: Four Essays*. Translated by Caryl Emerson. Edited by Michael Holquist. Austin: University of Texas Press.

Basso, Keith H. 1988. "'Stalking with Stories': Names, Places, and Moral Narratives Among the Western Apache." In *Text, Play, and Story*, edited by E. M. Bruner, 19–55. Washington D. C: American Ethnological Society.

Baynham, Mike. 2015. "Narrative and Space/Time." In *The Handbook of Narrative Analysis*, edited by Anna De Fina and Alexandra Georgakopoulou, 119–139. Malden, MA: Wiley Blackwell.

Berlivet, Luc, and Ilana Löwy. 2020. "Hydroxychloroquine Controversies: Clinical Trials, Epistemology, and the Democratization of Science." *Medical Anthropology Quarterly* 34 (4): 525–541.

Biehl, Joao. 2007. "Pharmaceuticalization: AIDS Treatment and Global Health Politics." *Anthropological Quarterly* 80: 1083–1126.

Black, Steven P. 2021. "Portable Values, Inequities, and Techno-Optimism in Global Health Storytelling." *Journal of Linguistic Anthropology* 31 (1): 25–42.

Briggs, Charles L., and Daniel C. Hallin. 2016. *Making Health Public: How News Coverage is Remaking Media, Medicine, and Contemporary Life*. New York: Routledge.

Brooks, Jennifer, Kristy Campbell, Bethel DiMaggio Ziesenitz, Jessica Doyle, Kathleen A. Ethier, Christine Hall, Cyndi Hatcher, Healther King Smith, Nancy Messonnier, Mark L. Messonnier, Mary Helen O'Conner, Daniel C. Payne, Rebecca Payne, Jessica Rogers Brown, Michele Russell, Michael Sauer, Kristen Sullivan, and Sarah Szlam. 2020. "Dear Decaturish – City Schools of Decatur Should Offer

In-Person Learning Option for All Students." *Decaturish*. Accessed 9/13/2022. https://decaturish.com/2020/12/dear-decaturish-city-schools-of-decatur-should-offer-in-person-learning-option-for-all-students/.

Brunson, E. K., M. Schoch-Spana, M. Carnes, D. Hosangadi, R. Long, S. Ravi, M. Taylor, M. Trotochaud, and T. G. Veenema. 2021. *Carrying Equity in COVID-19 Vaccination Forward: Guidance Informed by Communities of Color*. Baltimore, MD: Johns Hopkins Center for Health Security.

Carr, E. Summerson. 2010. "Enactments of Expertise." *Annual Review of Anthropology* 39: 17–32.

CDC. 2007. *Interim Pre-Pandemic Planning Guidance: Community Strategy for Pandemic Influenza Mitigation in the United States. Early, Targeted, Layered Use of Nonpharmaceutical Interventions*. Atlanta, GA: Centers for Disease Control and Prevention (U.S. Department of Health and Human Services).

Clarke, Adele E., Janet K. Shim, Laura Mamo, Jennifer Ruth Fosket, and Jennifer R. Fishman. 2003. "Biomedicalization: Technoscientific Transformations of Health, Illness, and U.S. Biomedicine." *American Sociological Review* 68 (2): 161–194.

Frank, Richard G., Leslie Dach, and Nicole Lurie. 2021. It was the Government that Produced COVID-19 Vaccine Success. *Health Affairs*. DOI: 10.1377/hblog20210512.191448 Accessed 08/04/2022.

Gavin, Kara. 2020. "Flattening the Curve for COVID-19: What Does It Mean and How Can You Help?" *Health Blog: University of Michigan Health*. August 11, 2022. https://healthblog.uofmhealth.org/wellness-prevention/flattening-curve-for-covid-19-what-does-it-mean-and-how-can-you-help.

Goldhill, Olivia. 2022. *Encouraged by Right-Wing Doctor Groups, Desperate Patients Turn to Ivermectin for Long Covid*. Edited by STAT. https://www.statnews.com/2022/07/26/ivermectin-has-become-a-popular-treatment-for-long-covid-with-a-push-from-doctors-with-ties-to-right-wing-political-groups/

Jones, Davis S., and Stefan Helmreich. 2020. "The Shape of Epidemics." *Boston Review*, June 26, 2020.

Li, Nan, and Amanda L. Molder. 2021. "Can Scientists Use Simple Infographics to Convince? Effects of the 'Flatten the Curve' Charts on Perceptions of and Behavioral Intentions toward Social Distancing During the COVID-19 Pandemic." *Public Understanding of Science* 30 (7): 898–912.

Lovelace Jr., Berkeley, and Kevin Breuninger. 2020. Trump Says He Takes Hydroxychloroquine to Prevent Coronavirus Infection Even Though It's an Unproven Treatment. *CNBC*. https://www.jsonline.com/story/news/politics/2022/08/24/trump-advisors-turned-ron-johnson-push-hydroxychloroquine/7886363001/ Accessed 08/04/2022.

Moyer, Eileen, and Vinh-Kim Nguyen. 2016. "Is the 21st Century the Age of Biomedicalization?" *Medicine Anthropology Theory* 3 (1): i–vii.

Ochs, Elinor. 2004. "Narrative Lessons." In *A Companion to Linguistic Anthropology*, edited by Alessandro Duranti, 269–289. Malden, MA: Blackwell Publishers.

Ochs, Elinor, Patrick Gonzales, and Sally Jacoby. 1996. "When I Come Down I'm in a Domain State: Talk, Gesture, and Graphic Representation in the Interpretive Activity of Physicists." In *Interaction and Grammar*, edited by Elinor Ochs,

Emanuel Schegloff and Sandra A. Thompson, 328–369. Cambridge: Cambridge University Press.

Press, Associated. 2021. "In CDC's Backyard, School Reopening Debate Divides Experts." *WABE.org*. Accessed 09/13/2022. https://www.wabe.org/in-cdcs-backyard-school-reopening-debate-divides-experts/.

Pritchard, Duncan. 2007. "Recent Work on Epistemic Value." *American Philosophical Quarterly* 44 (2): 85–110.

Rapp, Rayna. 1998. "Refusing Prenatal Diagnosis: The Multiple Meanings of Biotechnology in a Multicultural World." *Science, Technology and Human Values* 23 (1): 45–70.

Ricoeur, Paul. 1984. *Time and Narrative*. Chicago, IL: University of Chicago Press.

Storz, Lauren, and Anna Wynfield. 2020. "How to Sense a Pandemic: Curves, Models, and the Affective Allure of Flattening." In *Pandemic Diaries: Affect and Crisis. American Ethnologist Website*, May 20, 2020, edited by Carla Jones. https://americanethnologist.org/online-content/collections/affect-and-crisis/how-to-sense-a-pandemic-curves-models-and-the-affective-allure-of-flattening/

Taylor, Janelle S. 2003. "Confronting 'Culture' in Medicine's 'Culture of No Culture'." *Academic Medicine* 78 (6): 555–559.

Wen, Leana S. 2021. "The Vaccine Success Story Needs to be Told." *The Washington Post*. https://www.washingtonpost.com/opinions/2021/04/20/covid-19-vaccines-are-an-extraordinary-success-story-media-should-tell-it-that-way/

Wolfgram, Matthew. 2016. "Science Talk and Scientific Reference." *Annual Review of Anthropology* 45: 33–44.

6 Recruiting Epistemic and Ethical Values for Global Health Audiences

Steven P. Black and Gabriela Alvarado

I (S. Black) first met Dr. Díaz in a coffee shop in Decatur, Georgia, in December of 2016. Díaz—a Costa Rican who had worked in global health for several years—was in Atlanta to advertise new education options offered by his Costa Rican non-profit organization (NPO), the Latin American Global Health Collective (LAG). Specifically, he was traveling to recruit US global health academics to create study abroad courses with LAG. This chapter's co-author, Gabriela Alvarado (who was a Costa Rican MA student at Georgia State University at the time), had convinced me to meet with her colleague. I was curious about whether meeting with Díaz could inform my new project on global health discourses. Since I was working from home on the day of our meeting, I asked if he and Alvarado could come to my favorite nearby coffee shop. The shop was a hipster café where many Emory students and faculty came to work, complete with comfy chairs, free Wi-Fi, shiny dark countertops, and overpriced specialty drinks and pastries. Díaz arrived armed with glossy folders and pamphlets branded with LAG logos and pictures, prepared to pitch his programs just as he had with other professors in Atlanta and other US cities. During his US tour, Díaz was not as successful as he had hoped. This prompted LAG leaders to start a website redesign process to attract professors and students and better represent the organization.

This chapter is about the LAG website redesign process in its broader sociocultural, historical, and linguistic context. While Costa Rica may seem far from Atlanta both spatially and conceptually, it is perhaps not so distant from key topics as it might feel at first. Though much of the communication discussed in this chapter happened online among participants located in Costa Rica, that communication was oriented primarily toward an imagined audience of US global health academics and students. This chapter's analysis of the website redesign process, in which the organization recalibrated its story and vision, offers insights about (1) the perspectives of US-based global health academics, (2) the sorts of training that global health students receive when they travel abroad (now considered

DOI: 10.4324/9781003561019-6

an important, if not essential, part of global health education), and (3) the role of nationality, wealth, and power differentials in the reproduction of inequities in global health. Additionally, this chapter provides an example of part of the online storytelling process that appears in the rest of this book only through interviews—the process of planning and creating online content. Finally, the chapter showcases the economic challenges that global health professionals may face when they attempt to deviate significantly from the sorts of techno-optimistic plots described in the previous chapters even while retaining the core epistemic and ethical values often associated with those plots.

While the previous chapters in this book have examined how global health professionals tell stories in various recorded and face-to-face contexts, including contexts that may be made available to audiences on websites, this chapter takes this analysis a step further to think about the ways that websites themselves can be conceptualized as stories. Verbally constructed stories are emplotted through the juxtaposition of temporally distinct social activities and events—often accompanied by the deployment of other semiotic resources—to suggest an implicit theory of how and why social activities and events are causally linked. Analagously, websites juxtapose key phrases, visual elements, and symbols in ways that similarly suggest causal linkages to craft an incipient story. In this chapter we draw from theorizations of commodification and mediatization, placing these two concepts in dialogue with linguistic anthropology scholarship introduced in Chapter 4 on audiences and audience design, to examine the process of creating one such story.

Raison D'Etre

By September 2017, the new LAG website, Facebook page, and Instagram account were up and running. LAG had been formed in 2015 by a team of Costa Rican health professionals. Most of these founding members, including its leader, Dr. Díaz, had been mentored by a Costa Rican medical visionary named Dr. Hernandez. Over decades of work, Hernandez developed a human rights and health equity approach that adapted the socialized Costa Rican healthcare system to meet the needs of marginalized Indigenous populations in southern Costa Rica.

In 2017, LAG created and posted a Facebook video titled "LAG—Raison D'Etre" (reason for being). All of LAG's online content, including this video, was in English—one indication that the main audience for the content consisted of American academics and students. The video featured inspirational orchestral music professionally edited to match a slide show, short descriptive texts, and visual transitions (e.g., crossfades). A script for the video was created by Gabriela Alvarado in consultation with Dr. Hernandez. In writing this script, Alvarado drew upon participant observation with LAG, including extensive conversations among LAG leaders during the organization's website redesign process. She also relied on her own background and expertise as a Costa Rican medical doctor who had practiced in rural Costa Rica, earned an MpH, and worked as a global health intern with an Atlanta-based NPO (Alvarado has since earned a PhD and works in health policy).

In the LAG Facebook video, a narrator voices the script that Alvarado wrote:

> The overall health of humans as shown by life-expectancy has increased dramatically worldwide, due to scientific and medical advances, as well as key public health policies. Unfortunately, severe disparities persist due to structural and socio-economic inequities ... It is imperative to train dynamic health professionals who are equipped to deal with the complexity of health issues today. This is the driving force that led to the creation of the Latin American Global Health Collective. At LAG, we believe health professionals should be educated and empowered to mobilize knowledge, and to engage in critical thinking that can facilitate ethical, sustainable, and population-centered approaches to health. We invite you to join us, and develop this new educational model that promotes a new type of health professional, one that can empower communities, enhance human well-being, and improve health around the globe. LAG. Transforming health education. Redefining health.

While this script deploys some of the techno-optimistic building blocks described in Chapter 5, it also departs from them in important ways. While the narrator describes "scientific and medical advances" (the "what we've done/what we're doing" building block), this is immediately followed by mention of some of the antiheroes described in Chapter 5 (e.g., public health policies and structural and socioeconomic inequities). Rather than simplifying global health solutions to a technological silver bullet, this narrative emphasizes the "complexity of health issues." The voice-over points toward the ethical value of caring for those who are unable to care for themselves, while also using key terms such as "critical thinking," "ethical, sustainable, and population-centered approaches," and "transforming health education," terms which match those that appear on the LAG website. And the narrative ends on an optimistic note with a discussion of how a "new type of health professional" will be capable of empowering communities, enhancing human well-being, and improving health around the globe (note the spatial generalization of "around the globe").

The video also features some of the multimodal poetic elements of liable and empowering affect described in Chapter 3, including images of

Indigenous Costa Ricans paired with an ostinato "sus chord" to provide an inspirational-sounding musical accompaniment. These images and sounds were carefully crafted to create a digital presentation of LAG's organization that could appeal to audiences of US university professors and students.

After receiving a version of this video created by professional Costa Rican video editors in mid-July 2017, Dr. Díaz showed the finished product to Alvarado. Alvarado mentioned that the narrator was speaking English with an accent associated with Latin American Spanish. She felt that some US students and professors might not take the Spanish-accented video, and thus the organization, seriously. Several years of living and working in Atlanta as a Spanish-dominant bilingual speaker had led Alvarado to an embodied knowledge of mainstream US interpretations of Spanish-accented English—interpretations that included harmful false stereotypes of Spanish speakers (see Rosa 2016 on raciolinguistic ideologies and Spanish in the United States). Upon hearing Alvarado's concerns, Díaz responded, "we should be proud of being Latin," and "the accent is like a badge of honor." A few minutes later, another Costa Rican LAG collaborator, Javier, viewed the video. Javier provided a few critiques and mentioned that some of the speaker's words were hard to understand. Despite these concerns, Díaz posted the video to Facebook.

The linguistic and other semiotic content of this promotional video illustrate LAG's efforts to attract academic audiences who might later enroll in the NPO's educational programming. These elements of the video aligned LAG with US-based global health discourses, while Díaz's insistence on a Spanish-accented voice-over was part of his resistance to what this effort may have otherwise indicated about LAG's relationship with the United States—namely, that LAG might be implicated in power structures involved in the reproduction of the very same inequities that Díaz hoped to combat through his organization.

Díaz hoped to help decolonize global health through his work; yet he had discovered that to do so, LAG needed a sustainable financial model. Pharmaceutical companies from high-income countries who donate to global health initiatives do well by doing good. In other words, these companies find financial success while doing something perceived to be ethical. Working with marginalized communities in a middle-income country, Díaz hoped to mirror this process and do good by doing well. He had first organized his NPO around health interventions and research. However, he soon realized that in order to contribute to the health and well-being of marginalized communities (through health interventions and research) he first needed to have the funds to do so. LAG hoped to find financial stability through global health educational programming.

In this attempt, LAG was enacting a financial model similar to other NPOs, but with academics rather than philanthropists as primary audiences for public-facing communication. Whereas the global health organizations discussed in previous chapters obtained funding by attracting donors through the circulation of stories that showcased their epistemic and ethical values, LAG obtained funding by attracting professors and students through the circulation of stories that showcased their ability to teach those values. In order to do so, LAG needed to be more explicit in articulating those values. Still, there is a great deal of overlap between these processes. Alvarado's participant observation in the website redesign process provided us with data on the sorts of conversations that may occur in many different global health (and other) NPOs as they design communications strategies to make their work both ethical and financially sustainable. At the same time, LAG was part of but at the margins of global health efforts and global health education in high-income countries.

A Note on Methods

In this chapter, we focus especially on LAG's creation of its global health education website, including our observations of LAG before, during, and after a meeting conducted on Skype. This involved adapting existing qualitative methods to non-typical situations. For instance, Black conducted an interview with Dr. Díaz over Skype, and Alvarado conducted participant observation during a website design meeting on Skype. Indeed, the website design meeting occurred with all participants on Skype on June 23, 2017, the same day as the Skype interview conducted by Black. Meeting attendees did not consent to be audio recorded but agreed that Alvarado could take fieldnotes. Alvarado notated the contours of the conversation, which are thus reported here as indirect quotations.

Internet-facilitated fieldwork may still be atypical in anthropological research, but it is becoming increasingly common (Wilson and Peterson 2002; e.g., Gershon 2010). And internet-facilitated interactions are becoming quite ordinary in everyday life in Costa Rica, as in the United States and elsewhere. Many Costa Ricans, especially urban elites, use the multifaceted and multimodal WhatsApp to communicate via cell phone. LAG leaders engaged in many work activities over Skype and WhatsApp as they traveled the country and the world. These apps afforded different types of engagement across time and space in ways that are increasingly familiar to many people (see Calhoun 2019: 31 on affordances of apps and online discourse genres). Our use of these media for research mirrored LAG's use of them for everyday work. Similarly, our interest in the LAG website's content followed students, professors, and administrators' engagement with the website as a point of entry into LAG's educational programming and recruitment.

Key Concepts: Commodification and Mediatization

In this chapter we use the concepts of commodification and mediatization to understand how website design can be central to the management of the interface between epistemic, ethical, and economic values in global health. Chapter 5 introduced a key perspective on commodification, describing it as a process that strips an entity of existing social connections (see Faudree 2020 on semiotic stripping). Significantly for this chapter, education has been described as a form of gift giving that tends to exceed this capacity of commodification (which may be why long-lasting relationships are so often formed through teaching and other forms of paid mentorship) (Tsing 2013: 23).

During commodification, particular qualities of an entity are identified and (re)evaluated in order to determine the entity's monetary value (Graber 2023). It is not immediately obvious which qualities of global health study abroad programs are evaluated in their commodification. It is true that students receive important knowledge through coursework (in good programs such as the ones run by LAG, at least). However, this can be learned in classroom contexts. It seems that what is most significant in study abroad programs is the ineffable experience of "being there" and the ethical sense of attunement to cultural difference that is assumed to result from that experience (especially in encounters with people from low-income communities). This becomes a significant component of the healthcare résumé. In other words, the thing that becomes valued and transportable via the résumé or CV—in other words, the thing that is commodified—is the encounter with cultural and socioeconomic difference in health contexts. This then becomes part of the study abroad participant's professional profile (and only then transportable in the sense that the participant themselves may move from job to job).

Before this commodified semiotic transfer can occur, though, first professors and administrators and then their students must be enticed to pay for and go on a study abroad trip. Websites and social media accounts are central tools for attracting these audiences—just as they are important tools for global health NPOs to attract donors. This chapter uses the concept of mediatization to understand this role played by websites. Mediatization is a linguistic anthropology concept that theorizes the "institutional practices that reflexively link processes of communication to processes of commoditization" (aka commodification; Agha 2011: 163). Previous research on mediatization, including research on public health (Briggs 2011), emphasizes that studying "the media" must also include tracing the complex ways that communicative patterns shift and morph (or stay the same) as they move from one context to the next, whether this may be online, in print, or in person. Broadly, this is the type of approach that has been taken throughout this book. In this chapter, we focus on how Dr. Díaz and his colleagues used LAG's website and Facebook page in their efforts to commodify their approach to global health by way of promotion of their study abroad programs.

Mediatization provides a theorization of how communication itself can be commodified—that is, how particular ways of speaking may come to have monetary value—and also how communication impacts the formation of other commodities. Mediatization may involve specification of "models of conduct—including models of 'communication'—designed to promote specific social practices" (Agha 2011: 163). LAG's study abroad programming helped to specify professional modes of conduct and genres of communication about care that were relevant for future global health professionals. In order to reach these students, though, LAG had to first attract professors and administrators to work with them. Analysis of LAG's website design process provides a window into the mediatization of global health values and details the sometimes-uncomfortable position of non-US health professionals in this process—uncomfortable in part because of LAG's efforts to commodify ethical values while simultaneously enacting them.

The Rise of Global Health Education

Given the rapid expansion of funding for global health over the past twenty years, it is no surprise that students in the global North who are pursuing health-related careers now find it desirable to have some sort of educational training in global health. Academic programs have proliferated to fill this new economic niche. This includes the creation of the NPO Consortium of Universities for Global Health (CUGH), an organization that is described as "a product of the expanding interest in global health."[1] Founded in 2008 with support from the Bill and Melinda Gates Foundation and later from the Rockefeller Foundation, CUGH later merged with the Global Health Education Consortium (founded in 1991 and focused more on health professional schools and residency programs). By 2023, CUGH included almost 200 member institutions located in forty countries and had recently hosted its fourteenth annual conference[2] (the academic conference being an important part of any field's scholarly bona fides).

As global health education has become institutionalized in university settings, it has made uneven progress in creating educational opportunities that reflect the core values of the field. One study conducted by global health educators explains,

> in spite of this demand-driven growth in the number of [global health] programs, breadth of opportunities, and amount of funding available to U.S. students, it has become apparent that our offerings do not

> consistently align with the priorities, needs, and preferences of our partners who generously host our trainees in the low- and middle-income settings that constitute the common global health destinations.
>
> (Adams et al. 2016: 1)

In other words, the socioeconomic relationship in global health education between low- and middle-income countries, on the one hand, and high-income countries, on the other, replicates and contributes to the socioeconomic relationship between these nations in global health as a whole.

Another study focused on undergraduate programming, working with eight undergraduate program directors affiliated with CUGH to review their undergraduate majors (Drain et al. 2017). Notably, one of the undergraduate programs surveyed was associated with an anthropology department and another with a multidisciplinary school that included anthropology (and study authors included an anthropologist). This study listed seven recommendations for undergraduate programs, including two related to study abroad courses: "facilitate and encourage experiential practicum and internship experiences" and "consider the risks/benefits of offering international experiences" (21–22). The risks of international experiences that the authors described include ethical concerns, and the authors encourage students looking for international experiences to "operate within the context of local needs and be aware of their own limitations, competencies, and skills" (Drain et al. 2017: 22). This risk of developing international programs that end up being extractive or exploitative of marginalized, low-income communities is not hypothetical, but rather historical. A pervasive problem for health education in particular has involved medical students and doctor-volunteers not considering their impact on marginalized communities and not understanding the significance of cultural difference during their educational experiences (Crump, Sugarman, and (WEIGHT) 2010; Sullivan and Berry 2017).

Costa Rica as a Global Health Training Ground

Increasingly, American university study abroad programs are being offered as short-term courses, consisting of quick trips to other countries for a few weeks or even less, and are being designed to include many activities that resemble tourist activities (Barkin 2018). Due to Costa Rica's reputation as a tourist-friendly tropical nation (Christian 2013), the country has become a destination for global health education programs. In this context, LAG and Costa Rica more generally play a complicated role in ongoing processes of the legitimation of global health. Costa Rica is a middle-income country with a robust socialized medical system (Clark 2002). By many measures, health outcomes in Costa Rica match or outpace those in the

United States. Still, common US stereotypes of Latin American countries—and Spanish speakers—as impoverished and in need of health interventions make the nation appealing to many as a site for service learning and education about cultural difference. Costa Rica's political stability allows for this education to take place in a low-risk environment, while its small per capita income in comparison with the United States yields a relationship of inequity in which US-based educators and students are providers of capital and Costa Ricans are recipients. LAG leaders were positioned in the middle of these relationships, relatively privileged in Costa Rica yet relatively marginalized with respect to most US academics.

Social scientists have expressed concerns about what students are actually learning on such programs around the globe (Bennett 2012). LAG wanted to respond to these concerns while also capitalizing on burgeoning student/professor and institutional interest. One of LAG's goals was to provide short-term study abroad experiences in a manner that socialized students into ethical perspectives and also directed attention and, in theory, resources to marginalized communities in Costa Rica. In 2018, LAG led over nine short-course programs in collaboration with professors employed by a wide range of institutions, from state commuter schools and research-intensive public universities to elite private colleges that are established leaders in global and public health. The following year, they led even more programs. US students came from across the socioeconomic spectrum, but the majority were white and middle or upper class. Many paid for these programs themselves, though a number were able to secure scholarships and fellowships. Students from elite institutions often had greater access to sources of funding.

The LAG Website Redesign Process

When LAG was first created in 2015, its primary mission had been to provide care to marginalized communities—especially Indigenous Costa Rican groups—by facilitating connections between global health professionals and members of these communities. By 2017, however, Díaz realized that this was not a financially sustainable model for the organization. LAG had not been able to secure enough funding through philanthropic means to continue with their existing plan. Díaz and his colleagues decided to start shifting the organization's focus toward global health education. As part of this shift, Díaz hired a communications consultant named María. María had a bachelor's degree in graphic design and previous experience helping to redesign professional websites. She spoke with Díaz and examined the existing LAG website. She then told Díaz (in Spanish), "you've got great ideas, but you are terrible at communicating them." This evaluation led LAG to begin the website redesign process.

At one point during the process, Díaz and María discussed using google analytics to track website traffic but did not follow up on this. They used a search engine optimization (SEO) process with keywords to make sure that audiences would be able to find the website. We do not have access to the list of keywords that were initially offered. However, the key phrases and design elements that eventually appeared on the finished LAG website were repeated in glossy advertising pamphlets that were given to potential participants and enrolled students. These elements were also reproduced in six-foot-tall portable full-color posters prominently displayed during their LAG courses. The act of carting heavy, space-occupying posters and stands around to remote parts of southern Costa Rica and exhibiting them during study abroad activities was demonstrative of the significance that LAG leaders placed on these images and texts as marketing devices and indexes of the organization's professionalism. Similar to the ways that the YouTube videos of other global health organizations were envisioned as a way to circulate shared narratives (a shared vision for an organization's employees), key phrases and concepts from the LAG website were also recontextualized in the ways that LAG leaders spoke to students and professors. While we cannot say how successful the website redesign in particular was in shifting the organization's ability to commodify educational offerings, LAG's nine study abroad programs in 2018 suggest that the overall effort was successful.

Study Abroad Decision-Makers as Key Audiences for the Circulation of LAG Stories

LAG's website was created in tandem with preparations for an official launch event, which would include an electronic press kit and a brochure. The Facebook video that we discussed at the beginning of this chapter was shown at the launch event. An article that was written about the event, which was published in a nationally circulating Costa Rican newspaper, featured a photo of four attendees: a dentist/professor associated with an Ivy League school of global health who was in Costa Rica to finalize and sign a collaboration agreement between LAG and the school; the president of a US-based philanthropic foundation that provided funding for the creation of LAG; the vice president of Costa Rica (Ana Helena Chacón); and Dr. Díaz. The photo provides a snapshot of a range of potential audiences for LAG's new website content—medical professionals from prestigious US institutions, donors associated with NPOs, and Costa Rican government officials, among others.

One of the questions that had to be answered during the organization's website design meeting was which of these (and other) possible audiences would be a central target for online content. This was discussed by participants in the meeting, including Díaz, communications consultant María, another web developer, and Alvarado, who was doing participant observation as a copyeditor on the project. This is how the meeting progressed.

It is June 23, 2017. Early in the meeting, María asks the group to define LAG in one minute. In response, Díaz stands up to deliver an "elevator pitch," which goes something like this (all quotations of discourse during this meeting are reconstructed from Alvarado's notes):

> Lo que es el LAG es una interfase entre nosotros, las comunidades, y las universidades en el extranjero para que puedan venir a tener experiencias inmersivas en el campo de la salud global y estas experiencias toman muchas formas, colores y sabores, como investigación, cursos, pasantías y prácticums.
>
> Translation: What LAG is, is an interface between us, the communities, and the foreign universities so that they can come to have immersive global health experiences in the country, and these experiences have many forms, colors, and flavors, such as research, courses, internships, and practicums.

Here, Dr. Díaz articulates a vision of LAG as an international educational coordinator. It is notable that he focuses on the idea of "immersive experiences," a concept that closely corresponds with a trend in short-term global health study abroad programs to commodify the very act of being in a place—especially a place marked as culturally and/or socioeconomically distinct from middle-class US contexts. Framing LAG's identity in this way helps to forge links with US-based education discourses. In this elevator pitch speech, Dr. Díaz also provides an initial profile of the audiences for the new website—people associated with foreign universities, including researchers, professors, and students.

Soon afterward, Díaz follows up by asking (in Spanish), "We already know who we are. Now who is our intended audience?" Continuing on this theme, he explains,

> Al comienzo eran estudiantes, ahora es el profesor que viene ... Nuestro mercado es la universidad; los que nos contrata es la universidad; al que tenemos que impresionar es al tomador de decisiones.
>
> Translation: At the beginning [the audience] was students, now it is the professor who comes... our market is the university; those with whom we contract are the universities; the ones that we need to impress are the ones who make the decisions.

Here, Dr. Díaz articulates not only his understanding of potential website audiences but also his previous experience with the process of running study abroad programs. While there are non-profit and for-profit organizations that directly recruit students, Dr. Díaz had found that it was more feasible to recruit professors who would then create programs through their own universities. This was the result of his astute analysis of the process through which university study abroad courses are created. In the new model, LAG would work as a collaborator and facilitator, providing much of the course content and handling logistics of travel and study in Costa Rica. Since LAG would not be directly enrolling students, its main goal would be to appeal to professors who could recruit students from their universities and create programs that would yield course credits for the students. In this exchange, Díaz uses economically oriented terminology such as "our market" and "those whom we contract," supporting the idea that he sees generating interest, and ultimately income, as a primary purpose of the new website.

From Collaborative Development to Formative Programs

Whereas the global health NPOs discussed throughout this book often orient their websites such that their stories circulate among potential donors, in the Skype meeting, LAG decided to orient its website toward university professors and administrators. This was not a switch that Díaz took lightly. His examination of markets, contracts, and key decision-makers had evolved over the course of several years and represented a significant departure from the passion for providing care that had guided Díaz's career up to that point. He had come to the field of global health through medical training and his early work with his mentor in southern Costa Rica. In the process of and after attaining his medical degree, Díaz participated in a number of field medicine excursions in Latin America and east Africa. In my (Black's) interview with him on June 23, 2017, Díaz explained that these excursions had taught him that "multilateral agencies were the enemy." This was a similar sentiment to those I discussed in Chapter 3 when examining the ethical value of effectiveness and the emphasis that global health professionals place on public-private partnerships. Like the former CDC employee interview recounted in that chapter, Díaz had experiences in Latin America and East Africa that led him to the conclusion that multilateral agencies such as United Nations Programme on HIV/AIDS (UNAIDS) and WHO were too slow, too tied to bureaucratic processes, and too self-serving.

In response, in 2015 Díaz implemented the concept of "collaborative development" to form LAG with the goal of positively impacting health outcomes in southern Costa Rica. Following in the footsteps of their mentor, LAG leaders designed the non-profit to be primarily oriented toward Indigenous Ngöbe-Buglé communities who live both in and outside of

Indigenous territories in the mountainous Brunca region of southern Costa Rica. LAG was also meant to be oriented toward Panamanian Ngöbe migrants who live in a large Indigenous territory in Panama and cross the border into Costa Rica seasonally to work as coffee pickers. The NPO's creation and its purpose were rooted in the ethical imperative to care for these marginalized groups.

The organization began with three components: (1) providing formative programs and courses—referring to educational experiences related to global health; (2) facilitating academic research projects in the region; and (3) providing a "platform for collaborative development," as Díaz put it, with LAG organizing and aligning multiple regional NPOs and state-funded initiatives around common agendas. In other words, LAG was designed to be similar to many of the Atlanta-area NPOs discussed in earlier chapters—as an organizer of collaborators/partners.

When LAG was founded, this third component was meant to be its primary activity. However, the emphasis on collaborative development was not yielding enough funding. In our interview, Díaz explained,

> That little third component is one that we started with, actually, but then as time went by this little third component was not creating any revenue for us, so we decided to kind of flip the model around and start with the educational component, that we knew can create revenue in order to support the other components.

Díaz's concern with the creation of revenue, or lack thereof, through provision of care to marginalized groups, demonstrates a core challenge faced by many global health organizations: how can money be found to pay for health interventions in under-resourced and marginalized communities? While this can be hard for any NPO, the fact that LAG was based in Costa Rica rather than in a high-income country global health center such as Atlanta, New York, or Geneva (Switzerland) may have played a part in the organization's difficulties. As has been discussed throughout this book, the dominant model is for global health organizers to be based in high-income countries, while global health implementers and direct provisioners of direct care are more likely to come from low- and middle-income countries. In our interview, Díaz explained that his solution to the lack of income was to shift the organization's focus toward global health education. The hope was that this would generate funding that might later yield research, long-term investment, and, eventually, care for communities in southern Costa Rica. In this way, the creation of a new LAG website was linked to Díaz's previous focus on improving marginalized Costa Ricans' access to health care, though less directly than in his previous vision for what LAG could be.

Managing Economic and Ethical Values through Transformative Learning

At the website design meeting, Díaz kept his previous LAG focus on equity in mind as he entered into the discursive world of US-based faculty-led short-term study abroad programs. In Costa Rica, a country that is slightly smaller in size than West Virginia and home to about five million people, global health education is manageably small and connected. In the years that LAG was first formed, for instance, Alvarado and Díaz had been in contact with at least three programs who marketed themselves to American students. One course presented itself as "surf and study," infused with recreational activities such as coffee and chocolate tours, sunset horseback riding, zip-lining (a common tourist activity where one is harnessed, attached to a long metal line, and uses gravity to move through the tree canopy at high speeds), and white-water rafting. Another, focused on public health courses and Spanish competency, also encouraged students to explore volcanoes and go zip-lining in their free time. A third worked to inspire "global citizens" to make a difference and then go home with a "changed soul" (note the emphasis on the student's transformation rather than communities in which the student might work). As they positioned themselves in comparison with such programs, LAG leaders hoped to create an image that attracted students and professors but avoided some of the pitfalls they saw as associated with these other programs—e.g., exoticizing and further marginalizing impoverished Costa Ricans such as residents of Indigenous territories.

In their discussion of how to create such a nuanced vision, Díaz and the others eventually turned to the concept of transformative learning. Earlier in the conversation, when the topic of key concepts and terms had initially arisen, María had emphasized, "no queremos que el centro transmita 'surf and study,' queremos que sea una cuestión educativa que cambia perspectivas" ("we don't want the center to transmit 'surf and study,' we want it to be an educational matter that changes perspectives"). In response, Díaz articulated the idea of transformative learning. María elaborated further—"el centro busca re-educar" (the center seeks to reeducate)—but she then emphasized that they needed to find a nicer word because "reeducating" sounded too strong. Later, when the web designer again mentioned the notion of a target audience, María returned to Díaz's term, stating, "yo creo que la palabra clave es transformación" ("I think that the key term is transformation").

This exchange reveals a tension between discursive patterns associated with the ethical values of global health and discursive patterns associated with the economic values of global health education. Potential program participants and organizers may not all have been prepared to critically engage with ethical issues in current scientific medical and global health practices. These individuals might have been attracted to the "surf and study" or "global citizens" type of study abroad programs. LAG leaders were critical of such educational approaches that were, in their analysis, extractive. However, LAG needed to attract interest to income. Their challenge was to craft an institutional image that represented not just the ethical value of caring for those unable to care for themselves but also the commitment to equity and structural change while doing so. However, they also needed to appeal to a wide array of students and professors. Dr. Díaz and the other meeting participants settled on transformative learning as a key concept that could satisfy these alternative and potentially oppositional framings. The result was a novel mediatization of the key term "transformational learning."

After the website meeting, María sent a "fill in a blank" template to Alvarado with categories such as "what we do," "why are we different," and "our impact model." In her capacity as copyeditor, Alvarado created content based on the design meeting outcomes and sent it back to María, who replied that the content was too long. Alvarado edited, then Díaz reviewed the content, inserting and deleting as he saw fit. This led to the final LAG homepage layout.

On the redesigned LAG homepage, the term "transformative" appears twice: as a symbol that indicates "transformative learning"; and in the "what we do section," with the text "ethical and transformative global health educational programming." These appearances of transformation occur alongside the concept of collaboration, which appears eleven times in the redesigned website. For instance, a section titled "our impact model" lists "collaborative approaches" as a core part of the model. This section also includes a number of epistemic values for global health such as "evidence-based policies," and the idea that successful "interventions" may be "replicated." LAG's inclusion of these terms associated with the epistemic and economic values of global health (discussed in Chapters 4 and 5) reduced the textual differences between LAG's website and that of other global health media, including other global health education websites. This alignment with core ethical and epistemic values of global health was central to the commodification that was constituted in the website.

Minding the Gaps

In designing the website content, Díaz and other LAG leaders had to attend to the ways that their content was similar to and distinct from that of other study abroad programs and global health discourses. Scholarship on storytelling and other types of verbal performance theorizes this process using the concept of intertextual gaps (Briggs and Bauman 1992: 149). This is part of a way of thinking about storytelling as a dynamic process in which storytellers are always in the act of reproducing and transforming genres and stories through each next moment of their storytelling practice. Here, the term text refers not just to written words but to any stable, conventionalized linguistic pattern, such that intertextual refers to how any next instantiation of a text relates to previous instantiations and conventions (Hodges 2015). When stories are repeated with efforts made to avoid any innovation or changes—despite the fact that each telling is necessarily distinct because no two contexts for the telling will be exactly the same—this is described as managing intertextual gaps (Briggs and Bauman 1992: 150).

When one navigates to the LAG homepage (accessed 01/08/2019), a slideshow plays that is accompanied by a written description: "The Latin American Global Health Collective (LAG) prepares leaders with the competencies required to give ethical, sustainable, and just solutions to the global and local health challenges of today and tomorrow." One of the slides features a quote (possibly from a student or professor), "a truly comprehensive experience." The website's emphasis on competencies and the idea of having "an experience" matches the trends in global health study abroad programs mentioned earlier in this chapter, while the descriptors ethical, sustainable, and just point toward key values for the organization and for global health in general.

Scrolling down the page, one encounters the question, "why are we different?" This emphasis on difference could be interpreted within a commodification framework—as an indication of why students should choose LAG rather than the competition. At the same time, the website's answer to this question again emphasizes the group's ethical values. It lists the following themes: health equity centered, reciprocity, local ownership, fostering south-south partnerships, long-term partnerships, and community inclusion. In this way, the website becomes a possible entry point for socialization into global health discourses even as it commodifies these discourses. It also uses LAG's ethical values as a way to differentiate the organization in the broader market of study abroad courses, effectively mediatizing those values.

While the images that appear with this text do not deploy racialized affect in the same way as the global health websites discussed in earlier chapters, some broad similarities in the images leave these LAG image open to a variety of interpretations. A slideshow on the homepage includes images of smiling and intent students, smiling Latin American women and children on a beach, and a person with a backpack (a student?) walking alongside a woman who is wearing a traditional Indigenous dress. Recall that liable affect racializes marginalized populations through processes of simplification and containment, while empowering affect allows for complex, nuanced interpretations that are conceptually associated with whiteness (Berg and

Ramos-Zayas 2015). The students do appear to come from a wide range of ethnic and racial backgrounds and there are no images where people from marginalized communities are presented as helpless or destitute. At the same time, the students appear in front of a computer and projected lecture slides in one image and with a fancy backpack in another (full of who knows what sort of equipment), suggesting at least the possibility of the deployment of liable affect (associated with the Latin American family and Indigenous woman) and empowering affect (associated with the students). In this way, the LAG website walks a fine line—avoiding many of the pitfalls of racialized affect but still aligning enough to resonate with other global health websites and study abroad programs. In other words, the website displays LAG's management of intertextual gaps with global health discourses in general, and global health education discourses in particular.

This is not meant as a criticism of LAG's choices. Indeed, I know of the challenges involved in such an endeavor from my own experiences attempting to create a study abroad program and attract students.[3] Rather, this analysis is meant to highlight how difficult it is to stray from the reproduction of dominant global health discursive patterns and remain financially afloat. When Dr. Díaz and other LAG leaders redesigned their website, they were making choices about how to manage the intertextual gaps between their new content and the conventions of global health storytelling. Sometimes decision-making was conscious and verbalized, as when the group rejected "surf and study" programs. Other times decision-making relied on group members' implicit understanding of the aesthetics and conventions of global health storytelling. The balancing act involved in this management of intertextual gaps allowed the group to maintain a sense of commitment to core ideals while also making the website content recognizable enough to appeal to professors and students deciding where to go on a study abroad program.

Websites as Mediatizations of Care

It is important to emphasize the fact that the choices made by LAG leaders were not solely motivated by financial concerns (and neither are other global health NPO decisions when designing websites). As the vignette that opened this chapter indicates, Díaz was deeply committed to forging meaningful links between low- and middle-income countries (in this case, southern Costa Rica) and high-income countries, and focused on students and professionals who were able to provide resources—or who would potentially be able to do so after the completion of their studies. In this indirect manner, Díaz and other LAG collaborators understood their efforts as part of care work itself. In other words, the website was not only a mediatization of a discourse of care but was also a mediatization of care itself.

In the LAG meeting, discussion about how to successfully commodify LAG educational programming was intently focused on who their audience would be. This matches the analysis in the previous chapter of the relationship between websites/other online content and donor audiences, and is similar to situations described in previous research on commodified communicative activities where a speaker's distinct understanding of the composition of their audience leads them to shift their communicative style (Bell and Gibson 2011; Bogen 1987). Indeed, one of María's jobs as a consultant was to prompt Díaz to attend to audiences in this way. In other words, she encouraged Díaz to examine LAG's mediated image in relation to potential audiences with the goal of more successful commodification. In the LAG website design meeting, a discussion about audiences helped to clarify to whom LAG was meant to appeal, so that the website content, look, and feel could be modified in an attempt to better attract those audiences. This would lead to the design and implementation of study abroad courses that would generate income. The team's discussion of key audiences was a prelude to the management of intertextual gaps; and if they were successful in these efforts, they would attract professors who would recruit students, thus training the attention of current and future global health professionals on marginalized communities in Costa Rica. Students would purportedly be "transformed" into people who not only understood the structural inequities inherent in the world economic system but also felt the moral imperative to redress such inequities. While a new website may seem far removed from the moral imperative to implement global health interventions, the website design and its textual focus were rooted in Díaz's nuanced analysis of the large-scale socioeconomic and historical factors shaping not only southern Costa Rica's global health scene but also health care in low- and middle-income countries in general.

Though there is not a one-to-one correspondence, this Costa Rican example provides an additional example showcasing why global health NPOs have such well-developed online profiles and website content. A similar mediatization of care is evident in the work that other global health professionals do, resulting in the content discussed in Chapter 4. The dilemma of how to create income in a context where there is not enough capital is a dilemma shared not only by educational non-profits but also by global health organizations in general. After all, they are trying to provide care to those who cannot pay for it themselves.

Surely, as the previous chapters have demonstrated, global health websites are significant in organizational storytelling efforts that are ultimately aimed at soliciting donations that will sustain the NPOs. Though this goal remains largely implicit as global health stories constitute epistemic values (such as generalizability, reliance on data and testing) and ethical values (such as effectiveness, partnership, and collaboration), it becomes more clearly articulated in the annual reports and claims about transparency that are explicitly described as being oriented toward donors. Still, for not only LAG but also the global health professionals and philanthropists discussed in previous chapters, the end goal is to "do good" by providing health care for those unable to provide care for themselves. The website redesign discussion overviewed in this chapter suggests that global health websites might also be conceptualized as part of these efforts to do good.

LAG began with the primary goals of providing care and facilitating collaborations to care for marginalized communities. However, the organization was ironically hampered by their relative proximity to communities in need of care. In the context of Costa Rica's per capita annual income of around $16,000-adjusted US dollars and a population of just five million people, LAG's ability to generate income through grants and donations in Costa Rica was limited in comparison with their US colleagues. The financial stability of the NPO required it to change its primary focus to global health education, but this stability came at the cost of further removing LAG from activities of care. However, educational programming was still supposed to impact care in the long run. The new website, with its emphasis on transformation, sustainability, and equity, was to become an entry point for the process of students and professors to learn about LAG's ethical values, which would continue during study abroad programs. Unfortunately, this work of mediatization pulled LAG further away from the organization's earlier efforts to provide care, thus structurally aligning LAG professionals more with US-based global health professionals.

Conclusion

In stories told verbally, e.g., in face-to-face settings, the temporal unfolding of verbs, subjects, and objects placed in a particular order, affixes indicating tense and mood, and, consequently, phrases indicating discrete events and activities fit together to offer an implicit theory of how different moments of experience are causally linked. Techno-optimistic global health stories, in particular, offer a theory of how the past and present can be linked to an imagined future, describing novel technologies as heroes that will provide the ability to care for the world's most marginalized groups. Websites sometimes offer similar stories through recorded speech or written text, but the interactive, visual layout of a website also affords emplotment through other forms of juxtaposition such as the appearance of key words, phrases, or symbols in conjunction with images and links to other pages.

LAG's website redesign meeting was oriented toward crafting a story that would appeal to an audience of global health students and professionals of the global North, while at the same time attempting to integrate some of global health's antiheroes—equity and structural change—into the sorts of stories that this audience was already familiar with.

Our discussion of LAG's struggles and the role of the website design process in the resolution of these struggles has broader implications for understanding inequities in global health as a discipline, including the role of mediatization in the discipline's continuing development. As previously mentioned, it has been argued that what distinguishes global health from previous international health efforts is not so much new kinds of health-care interventions but rather new kinds of semiotic and semantic moves being made in defining what is "global" and what is "health" (Adams 2016; Brada 2011; Fassin 2012). Study abroad legitimizes aspiring US health professionals' résumés, helping a new generation on their career paths at US-based non-profits and government institutions by giving them "global" experience while simultaneously defining what that global experience may be.

One troubling aspect of this arrangement is the question of what happens to care in the process. This is similar to the concern mentioned by Paul Farmer (2023), who explains,

> Caregiving has been largely stripped out of public health, and nowhere is this more true than in the postcolony. Call this the myopia of the healthy and well placed, a staple of our current iterations of global health. Disease control is not at all the same as caring for those afflicted by pathogens, which like other pathogenic forces… strike some while others are spared.
>
> (xix)

For Díaz and other LAG leaders, care and caring is indirect, as it is for global health professionals in high-income settings such as Atlanta. Care manifests in the ability of these individuals and organizations to direct resources and programming for *other* organizations (usually those based in low- and middle-income countries). Though global health professionals may feel that they are enacting care by mediatizing core values, Farmer's retort emphasizes that this is not the same as working as a doctor or nurse in a resource-poor setting, because there is a level of abstraction and distance at play here. The final chapter of this book explores how this level of abstraction, alongside spatial and epidemiological generalizations, may be interconnected with challenges associated with creating global health stories designed to increase health equity.

Notes

1 https://www.cugh.org/about/history/. Accessed 8/8/2023.
2 https://www.cugh.org/about/member-institutions/members-a-z/. Accessed 8/8/2023.
3 In fact, I decided to create and run a study abroad program in part to gain first-hand experience (participant observation) about the creation and management of such a program.

References

Adams, Lisa V., Claire M. Wagner, Cameron T. Nutt, and Agnes Binagwaho. 2016. "The Future of Global Health Education: Training for Equity in Global Health." *BMC Medical Education* 16 (296): 1–7. https://doi.org/10.1186/s12909-016-0820-0.

Adams, Vincanne. 2016. "What Is Critical Global Health?" *Medicine Anthropology Theory* 3 (2): 186–197.

Agha, Asif. 2011. "Meet Mediatization." *Language and Communication* 31 (3): 163–170.

Barkin, Gareth. 2018. "Either Here or There: Short-Term Study Abroad and the Discourse of Going." *Anthropology and Education Quarterly* 49 (3): 296–317.

Bell, Allan, and Andy Gibson, eds. 2011. "Staging Language: An Introduction to the Sociolinguistics of Performance." *A Special Issue of the Journal of Sociolinguistics* 15(5).

Bennett, Milton J. 2012. "Paradigmatic Assumptions and a Developmental Approach to Intercultural Learning." In *Student Learning Abroad: What Our Students Are Learning, What They're Not, and What We Can Do About It*, edited by Michael Vande Berg, R. Michael Paige, and Kris Hemming Lou, 90–114. Sterling, VA: Stylus.

Berg, Ulla D., and Ana Y. Ramos-Zayas. 2015. "Racializing Affect: A Theoretical Proposition." *Current Anthropology* 56 (5): 654–677.

Bogen, James. 1987. "Finding an Audience." *IPrA Papers in Pragmatics* 1 (2): 35–65.

Brada, Betsey Behr. 2011. "'Not *Here*': Making the Spaces and Subjects of 'Global Health' In Botswana." *Culture, Medicine, and Psychiatry* 35 (2): 285–312.

Briggs, Charles L. 2011. "On Virtual Epidemics and the Mediatization of Public Health." *Language & Communication* 31 (3): 217–228. https://doi.org/10.1016/j.langcom.2011.03.003.

Briggs, Charles L., and Richard Bauman. 1992. "Genre, Intertextuality, and Social Power." *Journal of Linguistic Anthropology* 2 (2): 131–172.

Calhoun, Kendra. 2019. "Vine Racial Comedy as Anti-Hegemonic Humor: Linguistic Performance and Generic Innovation." *Journal of Linguistic Anthropology* 29 (1): 27–49.

Christian, Michelle. 2013. "'...Latin America without the Downside': Racial Exceptionalism and Global Tourism in Costa Rica." *Ethnic and Racial Studies* 36 (10): 1599–1618.

Clark, Mary A. 2002. "Health Sector Reform in Costa Rica: Reinforcing a Public System." *Woodrow Wilson Center Workshops on the Politics of Education and Health Reforms*. Washington, DC.

Crump, John A., John A. Sugarman, and The Working GRoup on Ethics Guidelines for Global Health Training (WEIGHT). 2010. "Ethics and Best Practice Guidelines for Training Experiences in Global Health." *The American Journal of Tropical Medicine and Hygiene* 83 (6): 1178–1182.

Drain, Paul K., Charles Mock, David Toole, Anne Rosenwald, Megan Jehn, Thomas Csordas, Laura Ferguson, Caryl Waggett, Chinekwu Obidoa, and Judith N. Wasserheit. 2017. "The Emergence of Undergraduate Majors in Global Health: Systematic Review of Programs and Recommendations for Future Directions." *American Journal of Tropical Medicine and Hygiene* 96 (1): 16–23.

Farmer, Paul. 2023. "Against the Grain: Medical Anthropology in the Anthropocene." In *Arc of Interference: Medical Anthropology for Worlds on Edge*, edited by João Biehl and Vincanne Adams, xi–xxi. Durham, NC: Duke University Press.

Fassin, Didier. 2012. "That Obscure Object of Global Health." In *Medical Anthropology at the Intersections*, edited by Marcia C. Inhorn and Emily A. Wentzell, 95–115. Durham, NC: Duke University Press.

Faudree, Paja. 2020. "'Making Medicine' with *Salvia divinorum*: Competing Approaches and Their Implications." *Medical Anthropology* 39 (7): 582–596.

Gershon, Ilana. 2010. *The Breakup 2.0: Disconnecting O ver New Media*. Ithaca, NY: Cornell University Press.

Graber, Kathryn E. 2023. "Textures of Value: Tactility, Experience, and Exclusion in the Cashmere Commodity Chain." *Economic Anthropology* 10 (2): 186–196.

Hodges, Adam. 2015. "Intertextuality in Discourse." In *The Handbook of Discourse Analysis,* 2nd Edition, edited by Deborah Tannen, Heidi E. Hamilton and Deborah Schiffrin, 42–60. Hoboken, NJ: John Wiley & Sons, Inc.

Rosa, Jonathan. 2016. "Standardization, Racialization, Languagelessness: Raciolinguistic Ideologies across Communicative Contexts." *Journal of Linguistic Anthropology* 26 (2): 162–183.

Sullivan, Noelle, and Nicole Berry. 2017. "Good Intentions and Murky Ethics: How Anthropology Matters in Short-Term Global Health Travel." *Anthropology News* 58 (6): 11–13.

Tsing, Anna. 2013. "Sorting Out Commodities: How Capitalist Value Is Made Through Gifts." *HAU: Journal of Ethnographic Theory* 3 (1): 21–43.

Wilson, Samuel M., and Leighton C. Peterson. 2002. "The Anthropology of Online Communities." *Annual Review of Anthropology* 31: 449–467.

7 Reimagining the Future of Global Health Equity, and What This Says about Storytelling and Value

> What is important for the speaker about a linguistic form is not that it is a stable and always self-equivalent signal, but that it is an always changeable and adaptable sign.
>
> —V. N. Volsinov, *Marxism and the Philosophy of Language*, 68 (Volosinov 1973 [1929])

On the Bill and Melinda Gates Foundation website, a smiling African woman in a yellow, black, and white dress and turquoise and white headscarf holds her infant up for a picture. Though the background of the image is blurry, the outlines of a large thatch-roofed hut are visible in the distance. This image, which is a racialized index of care, accompanies a story published on August 21, 2018, by Ryan Bell (a "feature writer" for the foundation) titled "Under the Microscope: Learning More about Childhood Mortality."[1] The story begins with a history of the verbal autopsy in scientific medicine from 1665 onward. Verbal autopsy is a method for ascertaining a deceased person's cause of death by asking questions of caregivers who were close to them (e.g., family members). Bell explains, "Today, health researchers still rely on verbal autopsies—albeit with much improved protocols." The deputy director of surveillance and epidemiology of the Bill and Melinda Gates Foundation is quoted as saying, "But for specific infectious diseases, [verbal autopsies are] terrible. There's no way a mother can tell you if her child died from pneumococcus or respiratory syncytial virus (RSV)." This is a statement of a biomedicalized problem.

Bell describes what the organization is doing—but the organization in this instance is not the Bill and Melinda Gates Foundation, but rather CHAMPS (Child Health and Mortality Prevention Surveillance) Health (discussed in Chapter 3). Bell explains that CHAMPS Health is going to use minimally invasive tissue sampling (MITS) to "extract tiny biopsies from the organs of deceased children." He also says that MITS samples are sent to both "the local laboratory and the Center for Disease Control in

DOI: 10.4324/9781003561019-7

Atlanta, Georgia," and notes, "The project, supported with a $75 million grant from the Gates Foundation, aims to diagnose cause of death at a microscopic level." Then he points to a hopeful future and a technological solution, quoting Dr. Shabir Madhi, who is the director of the CHAMPS site in South Africa. Dr. Madhi explains,

> For us to make the next leap, in terms of deciding what interventions need to be prioritized... we need to know: Why is it, in 2016, we still have five million children dying? What are the causes? Which are the bacteria? Which are the viruses?

This story—and its appearance on a donor website—encapsulates the key ideas that I have discussed throughout this book. It provides an example of how core ethical and epistemic values of global health storytelling are constituted in stories through multimodal poetics and emplotment. But perhaps most significantly, it is evidence of how story circulation impacts the economics of the field. This narrative is closely connected with the CHAMPS Health video analyzed in Chapter 3. In fact, from a linguistic anthropological perspective the two might be said to be recontextualizations of the *same* story. The appearance of the story on the Bill and Melinda Gates Foundation website demonstrates one reason why philanthropists care about and even make funding decisions based on the sorts of stories that particular NPO (non-profit organization) leaders tell about their organizations' work. They do so because when donors give money to NPOs, NPO stories become philanthropists' stories.

The semiotic model of commodification and gift giving that I discussed in earlier chapters explains the function of this story transfer. Recall that commodification strips an entity of social values (the connections of something to the social relationships in which it was produced or exchanged), thus making that entity capable of being assigned a monetary value. The Gates Foundation website demonstrates how the reverse happens in global health philanthropy: social meaning is assigned to the exchange of money or other commodified resources. And a key part of how this social meaning is assigned is the recontextualization of an NPO story.

But there is also something more at stake. When NPOs tell future-oriented stories, they are not only imagining the future of global health into being but also staking out claims about actions they will take. In this way, the ever-present audience of potential donors shapes global health's goals and future actions. And when global health professionals tell techno-optimistic stories to attract donors, they limit the amount of attention the field pays to structural inequities–inequities that have very clear impacts on the health of communities. In this way, storytelling imaginatively (re)constitutes values while simultaneously limiting the scope of imagined futures (see also Kockelman 2020: 101–104).

The word "story" may have the connotation of not being a kind of action (as in "put your money where your mouth is"), or not being serious or true (as in "that's just a story"). In anthropology, the study of storytelling has sometimes been sidelined in favor of work that seeks to understand "big" questions about things like epistemology, ethics, and economics. However, in this book I have used the theoretical toolkit of linguistic anthropology to reveal how stories are actually central to these big questions—not only in the *display* of epistemic, ethical, and economic values but also in the *constitution* of these values (how these values are imagined into being). Multimodal poetics play a key role in constituting affect, allowing storytellers to craft evaluative stances focused on what one could, should, or must do. Circulation (telling, retelling, and transforming stories) provides a means by which people create associations among distinct tellers, audiences, and values. Emplotment establishes connections between events and times, allowing storytellers to make causal claims that can then be projected into the future. And future-oriented stories, in particular, may shape future action. After all, an NPO storyteller who tells this sort of narrative (especially a person or organization that is then given funding) might be expected to do what they say they are going to do.

In this book I have argued that storytelling is an important part of how global health professionals constitute values and emplot future actions. It follows that changing the sorts of stories that global health professionals tell has the potential to shift not just the image of the field but also its socioeconomic organization. However, the degree to which global health storytellers can be innovative is limited because meaning-making is always a collaborative process shaped by both one's audience(s) and the existing socioeconomic relationships among performers and audiences. Still, there is always room for creative action. Drawing from the analysis of storytelling offered in this book, in this chapter I utilize recent scholarship about public and global health (e.g., Kerry et al. 2014; Yates-Doerr 2020; Briggs 2024) to suggest some specific, practical changes that can be made to global health stories (and thus to global health perspectives and values) to help these stories better align with global health professionals' stated interest in equity and decolonization. In the remainder of this concluding chapter, I discuss two key lessons for global health storytelling: lesson #1 is to broaden epistemic values, and lesson #2 is to reorient ethical values toward accompaniment. After examining both of these lessons, I take a step back to discuss how the analysis I have presented throughout the book contributes to the anthropological study of value and storytelling.

Lesson # 1: Broaden Epistemic Values

In this book I described the emplotment of epistemic values in public and global health with a special focus on the early part of the COVID-19 pandemic. The epistemic values of "data-driven" contemporary global health discussed here overlap significantly with those of scientific medicine in general—for instance, a reliance on randomized controlled trials and the use of laboratory testing. In contemporary public and global health, such epistemic claims to truth are paired with statistical data and epidemiological analyses (Adams 2016). In this context, I discussed how the promotion of ineffective treatments for COVID-19 (such as Ivermectin and hydroxychloroquine) utilized the same techno-optimistic plots as promotion of effective treatments. This analysis explains one reason why it may be ineffective for health professionals to simply argue that promotion of such ineffective treatments is "unscientific" without further qualifications—because stories about these treatments were also presented as being techno-optimistic and rooted in science. I also identified five key building blocks for the emplotment of techno-optimistic global health stories: (1) a statement of a biomedicalized problem; (2) a discussion of actions that have been taken, are being taken, or will be taken; (3) an emphasis on technology as a fix; (4) spatial and/or epidemiological generalization; (5) and projection to a hopeful future. My analysis suggests that global health storytelling could support equity in health interventions by expanding the scope of epistemic values in building blocks one, three, and four. This is not a critique of existing epistemic values, but rather a call to broaden the scope of those values in ways that recognize how health, socioeconomic structures, and culture are intertwined.

Include but do not limit the scope of identified problems to biomedicalized perspectives. The profound power of biomedicalization lies in its ability to identify, name, and treat illness in individual human bodies (Rabinow and Rose 2006). However, this individualization of illness often comes at the expense of a broader viewpoint of not only how but also why pathogens move through the world along particular pathways, infecting some but not others. For instance, the problem of infant mortality in low-income countries could be conceptualized not just in terms of individual exposure to particular pathogens to be named, identified, and treated, but also in terms of the physical (and environmental) living and working conditions that make low-income communities more likely to be exposed to the pathogens and for pathogens to spread more quickly through them.

Emphasize technological fixes, but also consider simpler challenges to the socioeconomic status quo. Taking a broader viewpoint does not mean supplanting of technology as a fix, but rather supplementing of technological fixes with interventions that impact socioeconomic structures. For instance, a careful consideration of infant mortality could include advocacy for a change to the conditions in which low-income individuals live and work (e.g., structural change to ensure access to clean water, food security, and health care).

Assume the ability to generalize spatially as a biological given but understand and respond to how specific cultural and historical contexts provide distinct contexts for the development of the health interventions. Too often, global health professionals start with a perspective that emphasizes the shared biological heritage of humanity (and thus the universal efficacy of treatments) and then see culture and history as barriers to the ability to enact a given intervention. For instance, a study conducted by CHAMPS Health about community perceptions of "minimally invasive tissue sampling" of deceased infants prior to the start of surveillance found significant "tension" in communities and identified religion as a primary source of tension, arguing that "Religious leaders in the communities where CHAMPS is working require time to understand the procedure and how it relates to their religious beliefs and practices" (Blevins 2019: S290). The anthropological approach that I am advocating in this book calls for a different sort of story during project development, one that describes meeting with community stakeholders such as religious leaders not after the project has been designed (as CHAMPS did) but during the process of designing it (which likely entails not designing these stories and projects in only in high-income settings); and meaningfully altering project parameters as advised by community stakeholders to increase the chances that a project will both succeed and contribute to the immediate health and well-being of communities (rather than only in some imagined future).

Beyond a Social Determinants Perspective

It is true that public and global health professionals already have a framework for broadening the scope of their epistemic claims: the social determinants of health. Now a core concept in public and global health, the WHO adopted the social determinants framework in 2005. At that time, the multilateral organization established a Commission on Social Determinants of Health, which operated from 2005 to 2008. The commission concluded with three large-scale recommendations: "1. Improve daily living conditions; 2. Tackle the inequitable distribution of power, money, and resources; 3. Measure and understand the problem and assess the impact of action."[2] There is not much evidence of uptake of any of these recommendations in public and global health.

Nonetheless, CDC has adopted the WHO's definition of the social determinants of health; CDC describes this as

> the nonmedical factors that influence health outcomes. They are the conditions in which people are born, grow, work, live, and age, and the wider set of forces and systems shaping the conditions of daily life.

> These forces and systems include economic policies and systems, development agendas, social norms, social policies, racism, climate change, and political systems.[3]

Especially given the way this concept has entered the public and global health mainstream, it is notable that it does not often appear even indirectly in the stories told by global health professionals in public settings (as I have analyzed in this book). For instance, in the CHAMPS story told on the Gates Foundation website, recall that a doctor asks, "Why is it, in 2016, we still have five million children dying? What are the causes? Which are the bacteria? Which are the viruses?" Why not also ask, "What are the living conditions that shape people's exposure to these viruses?" In contrast, a narrow biomedicalization of the causes of child mortality focuses on viruses and bacteria. It does not address social determinants of health by asking any questions about how pathogens come into contact with children in the first place—in impure water? due to environmental degradation?—or why these broader factors disproportionately affect poor and marginalized communities. In the Gates Foundation's narrative, the doctor's narrow biomedicalized viewpoint is not challenged or expanded.

While a necessary first step in such cases is to attend to and incorporate a social determinants perspective into global health stories, anthropologist Emily Yates-Doerr (2020) argues that even doing so may not go far enough. She explains,

> The social determinants framework may uphold and even exacerbate conditions of inequality by prioritizing and targeting a form of health that has been predetermined by distant experts. Its concern for justice and inequality has an inspiring ring; but its reliance on "determinacy" doesn't go far enough in challenging—and changing—the health care systems in which it operates. My concern is that the desire to address the roots of a pre-given problem imagined to begin at a measurable point and to then advance to a predictable (i.e., determinant) place, sets us on a path toward prescriptive solutions that do not result in the deep structural transformation they claim to inspire.
>
> (379–380)

In other words, as mentioned, broadening the scope of epistemic values should entail radically altering the design of interventions and centering the perspectives of those who are members of the communities that are targets of health interventions and adopting those community's definitions of health. In practice, whether in clinics or strategy meetings where interventions are being designed, this means creating what Charles L. Briggs (2024) has termed incommunicability-free zones, "spaces where confronting inequities does not promote hierarchies of knowledge or stigmatize some participants as being out of the loop, ignorant, or misguided" (93).

Bringing the insights of such revised practices of knowledge production and intervention design into global health storytelling might involve telling stories where "antiheroes" (here, structural interventions rooted in community concerns and goals) play leading roles. Here, the term antihero makes sense in the context of the dominant story plots favored by philanthropists in high-income countries. Whether an intervention is considered mainstream or alternative depends on the cultural and historical context in which the story is being told. Novel technological solutions may still have a role to play, but this may become more of a supporting role, depending on the situation and context. Here, a challenge for the field of global health is to restructure the design of projects to allow doctors, patients, and activists in low-income settings to take a leading role in creating future-oriented stories about the work that will be done. And a challenge for virtuosic global health storytellers in NPOs is to determine how to incorporate the insights of restructured project design into stories that will appeal to donors. Anthropologists can help with both of these challenges.

Juxtaposing Cultural-Economic-Historical Specificity with Biological Generalization

As the example of CHAMPS Health demonstrates, an additional concern for global health storytelling is how to juxtapose this radical centering of the perspectives—and thus also the specific cultural, economic, and historical context—of communities that are the targets for health interventions, on the one hand, with global health professionals' penchant for making broad biological generalizations (techno-optimistic plot building block four). In a spatial or epidemiological generalization, a technological fix is suggested to be applicable more broadly—either to other locations around the world or to other biomedicalized problems. NPO storytellers may frame an intervention in this way to showcase how funding for a particular intervention has the potential to have an even greater future impact on health, because the intervention could be applied in other contexts than the one in which an NPO is currently working.

Spatial generalization—moving from one particular socioeconomic and cultural context to a broader, perhaps universal applicability—is based on the fundamental tenet that all human bodies are broadly the same in biological terms. This idea, biological generalization, is a central component of 20th-century anti-racism. Indeed, anthropologists will be familiar with the common refrain that such a perspective can be traced back to the work of founder of US anthropology Franz Boas and his students, and/or to the work of underrecognized scholars of color from the same time period such as Anténor Firmin (Darnell 1998; Baker 2021; Fluehr-Lobban 2000). Such perspectives were developed in reaction to scientific claims of the time that race was rooted in biological differences. The basic stance of this form of anti-racism is of course that it is scientifically incorrect to associate differences in skin tone with differences in other characteristics, whether they be biological, social, or psychological characteristics. Much of this work emphasizes the idea that race is a social and linguistic construct—though one that has far-reaching consequences in a world where many nonetheless continue to turn to race as a way to understand human difference (Alim, Rickford, and Ball 2016; Rosa and Díaz 2020).

In scientific medicine, a central implication of humanity's shared biological heritage is the fact that a new medicine or vaccine that treats a disease for one group of should usually work for all people. It then follows that global health storytellers can generalize when projecting their work into the future—e.g., they can claim that a new technology or drug can be scaled up and offered in many different countries and settings. However, the reality is that efforts to generalize spatially tend to fall short, or at least are often hampered by the cultural, economic, and historical complexities associated with particular places and people. Sometimes, global health professionals respond to this by treating culture as a "barrier" to treatment (e.g., Nguyen 2008: 137). The anthropological perspective I am advocating shifts the responsibility for addressing this problem from target communities to global health organizations themselves, critiquing NPOs for cultural incompetency (Abramowitz, Marten, and Panter-Brick 2014: 11–12). In terms of global health storytelling, the science of biological generalization—the idea that human bodies are all similar in medically significant ways—needs to be paired with a counterpoint rooted in specificity, in the basic recognition of cultural, economic, and historical difference.

The need for just this sort of critical understanding of these contexts is described in a recent commentary published in the *Lancet Global Health* titled, "Time to Take Critical Race Theory Seriously: Moving Beyond a Colour-Blind Gender Lens in Global Health" (Yam et al. 2021). The authors of this piece argue that global health must attend to the intersection of race, gender, nationality, religion, and age in numerous overlapping contexts that include transnational "global racial ideologies and systems" but also "sociocultural and policy contexts within countries," community contexts, and project and organizational contexts (e389). Shifting global health storytelling practices in this regard should not be a herculean endeavor, given the fact that global health stories already emphasize the ethical values of partnership and collaboration. However, community leaders and other stakeholders must be allocated the power to help determine the scope of the questions asked in the design of health interventions, and global health must tell stories that valorize community-centered and community-specific solutions while still touting promise of applying novel medical treatments elsewhere with appropriate attention to each community's needs.

Lesson #2: Reorient Ethical Values toward Accompaniment

In Chapter 3 of this book, I discussed the multimodal poetics of ethical values, focusing on how concepts of effectiveness and collaboration are constituted in global health stories. While I presented collaboration—especially in public-private partnerships—as an ethical value, it is notable that global health's attention to equity and inclusion of voices and expertise from low-income communities that might be assumed to be central to this ethics often remains implicit. Rather, global health professionals tend to emphasize the significance of collaboration to effectiveness; and effectiveness is framed as an ethical value in the sense that being effective means pragmatically responding to the economics of global health and thus providing health care to the most people possible. In other words, collaboration and effectiveness are articulated within ethical frameworks oriented toward pragmatism and a "health for most" stance to providing care.

In Chapter 3, I also examined a significant problem in storytellers' use of the concepts of collaboration and effectiveness, namely, that they construct NPO collaboration and effectiveness using racialized affect. In global health videos and images, Blackness tends to be used to index care in ways that both rely on existing stereotypes and recreate them. While this trend has been noticeably declining over the past several years, the underlying premise remains: global health interventions are planned "here" (in high-income countries, where the majority of NPO professionals are white despite increases in diversity over the years) while global health interventions happen "there" (in low-income countries) (Brada 2011, 2017). A solution to the reorienting of ethical values is interrelated with earlier suggestions for how to broaden epistemic values by further centering the experiences and perspectives of patients, doctors, activists, and community members in communities that are the targets of health interventions. Luckily, a theoretical and storytelling framework already exists that does so, and it is a framework that is already known in academic global health: the model of accompaniment (mentioned in Chapters 3 and 4).

How to Tell Accompaniment Stories

When I had the opportunity to interview Dr. David Addiss (recall that he is a global health academic and practitioner with many years of experience at CDC, the Task Force for Global Health, and Emory University), I asked him whether or not he had "noticed any big changes over the past twenty years or so" in public and global health. Here is how he responded:

Interview with David Addiss on 12–6–2016 starting at 7 min 04 sec

> Addiss: I think if I were to say what's shifted—to me, it's starting to shift now, and I think it's also threatened—but the major trend that I see in global health is this articulation of interconnectedness, the values of solidarity and accompaniment that Paul Farmer and others have talked about...[lines omitted where Dr. Addiss mentions a few academic global health programs that enact solidarity in their work]... and yet what we're really talking about is academics. That kind of thinking and that kind of language has not seeped into the practice and funding of global health. But I think the future of global health lies in embracing that and then questioning the structures that are required to deliver that kind of solidarity.

As Dr. Addiss explains, while the theory of accompaniment is becoming better known in academic global health, "that kind of language has not seeped into the practice and funding" of the field. My analysis in this book suggests that shifting global health stories to draw from the concept of accompaniment could help lead the charge in such a change in practice and funding.

The concept of accompaniment emerged out of Latin American social movements and liberation theology. It has been adapted to a range of activities and settings (including research on language and culture—see Bucholtz, Casillas, and Lee 2016). Dr. Addiss' mention of Paul Farmer in particular makes sense because Farmer made it a central part of his life's work to develop and operationalize the idea of accompaniment in global health settings in the service of "supporting the poor on the road toward well-being, prosperity, peace, and—indeed—aid independence. It begins with listening to and learning from one's intended beneficiaries, and working alongside them until they deem a task completed" (Kerry et al. 2014: 487). This approach can be boiled down to eight core principles (Weigel, Basilico, and Farmer 2013: 294–296):

- Favor institutions that the poor identify as representing their interests
- Fund public institutions to do their job
- Make job creation a benchmark of success
- Buy and hire locally
- Co-invest with governments to build strong civil services
- Work with governments to provide cash to the poorest
- Support regulation of international nonstate service providers
- Apply evidence-based standards of care that offer the best outcomes

It is notable that there is not much in these principles that explicitly addresses cultural relativity or identification of cultural barriers to health interventions. On the other hand, in some ways attention to cultural difference pervades the entire approach, which is rooted in leadership by members of communities that are the targets of health interventions (meaning that these leaders will bring their cultural perspectives to a given intervention's design and implementation).

With a number of key collaborators including Jim Kim (discussed in Chapter 4), Paul Farmer turned accompaniment into a successful way to run a global health NPO called Partners in Health (PIH). A three-part YouTube video series about PIH's Haiti Cholera Vaccine Project showcases the organization's approach to global health storytelling.[4] These videos do not shy away from showing images of sick Haitians or impoverished communities but couple those images with videos of Haitian workers in local communities collecting data and administering vaccines. The phase two video also features an interview with a member of a target community who explains in her own words why the project is important to her. This centering of Haitian voices, perspectives, and actions is both a representation of the accompaniment approach that PIH has already enacted and also a model for future interventions.

In a featured video on the PIH YouTube channel posted in October 2023, PIH co-founder Ophelia Dahl talks about Paul Farmer's vision as part of a call for a "global day of action."[5] Much of her speech is edited to be a voice-over in conjunction with images of Farmer working in Haiti. Dahl says,

> When my friend Paul talked about global health, he often talked about failures of imagination. It wasn't that the best treatments didn't work for the poorest, sickest patients, or that world class hospitals couldn't be built in impoverished areas. It was a failure of imagination. A failure to imagine and pursue a world where all patients everywhere have access to the highest standard of care; a world where no patient died of a treatable disease or stayed sick because they couldn't afford care. Paul not only imagined this world; he dedicated his life to making it a reality.

In the context of my analysis in this book, it is notable that Dahl uses the framework of imagination—and explains that Farmer viewed problems in global health as failures of the imagination. Farmer imagined another way of doing global health into being. However, Paul Farmer was a uniquely talented and driven individual. PIH's use of his memory (he passed away in 2022) in creating stories for fundraising indicates that it might be difficult for other NPOs to replicate the organization's storytelling successes without Paul Farmer.

The ability to move beyond academic discussions of accompaniment and incorporate it into the design and implementation of health interventions would be aided by a reconsideration of techno-optimistic storytelling plot building block three (a discussion of actions that have been taken, are being taken, or will be taken). While it may be the case that in the future accompaniment will be a widely known term in global health discourses, in the short term when creating stories for potential donors it may make the most sense to broaden the existing ethical values of partnership and collaboration. This would entail emphasizing the central role of affected community members and target community health systems in the design of a health intervention.

A Note on Rethinking Economic Values

In Chapter 4 of this book, I described the values with which global health professionals approach the circulation of stories, with special attention paid to how the stories might circulate among donors. I focused on the role that the values of transparency, successfulness, and narrative virtuosity play in shaping storytelling. Global health NPOs aim to not just be transparent, but also to demonstrate and communicate this transparency to others. They want not only to be successful but also to present themselves as capable of success. And they approach both of these tasks through storytelling, valuing narrative virtuosity as a skill that helps their stories to circulate among global health professionals and donors. And as I discussed earlier in the conclusion, NPOs' tellings of these types of stories occur in a context where the stories become linked to the public persona of the philanthropists who donate to their organization. The economic framework that underlies these activities is neoliberal capitalism, a system that involves limited governmental spending and a reliance on NPOs to fill gaps in the provision of care.

In Chapter 4 and throughout the book, I have approached the analysis of global health storytelling with the pragmatism that characterizes global health professionals' own approach. From such a standpoint, there is not much that might be done to shift the economic values of global health in the context of the field's reliance on philanthropy for a significant portion of its funding. And as discussed, global health professionals themselves tend to valorize public-private partnerships and emphasize the flexibility that comes with non-governmental funding. At the same time, the prevalence of a few very large donors can impact the field when those philanthropists set their own agenda.

For instance, when the Bill and Melinda Gates Foundation decided to fund efforts to decrease child mortality, one of the key ways that they disbursed this funding was through grants. A 2011 announcement of thirty-five million dollars' worth of grants (one of many such announcements over the years by the foundation) was framed as seeking "to engage the world's most creative minds to work on scientific and technological breakthroughs for pressing global health and development challenges."[6] As one global health professional explained to me in an informal conversation, when the Gates Foundation makes such an announcement, many organizations write grants and reorient their work with the hope of being the recipient of some of these funds. In this way, it is not just NPOs such as CHAMPS Health who are actually selected to partner with the Gates Foundation that are influenced by a philanthropist's interests, but rather the field as a whole shifts its storytelling and grant writing in an attempt to gain access to the funding of such a large philanthropic organization. It is unclear how the field might address this issue without confronting the entire economic organization of the public health around the world, but it does seem that global health could benefit from rethinking how priorities for the field are set. In particular, it could further emphasize what has been described as health systems strengthening, examples of which include working with low-income nations' existing health institutions, as well as working with and—when relevant—training health professionals in low-income nations.

On the Significance of Storytelling to Anthropological Theories of Value

In addition to these implications of this book for the broadening of epistemic values, the reorienting of ethical values, and the rethinking of economic values in global health, my analysis also suggests a novel anthropological model of the role of storytelling in the constitution of value systems. In theorizing storytelling and value systems, I have synthesized approaches from economic anthropology and linguistic anthropology to demonstrate how emplotment, multimodal poetics, and circulation function together to constitute values and value systems. One anthropological way to think about value is as a kind of second-order desire—as "some way of assessing the relative desirability of different desires, such that an actor (or interactor) can determine which one to act (or interact) for" (Kockelman 2016: 46). The anthropology of value theorizes how value makes actions meaningful by placing them in the context of a "larger social totality" (Graeber 2001: vii). Here, linguistic anthropological approaches can provide details on how, precisely, this semiotic process of meaning-making occurs (Kockelman 2020; Graber 2023; Shankar and Cavanaugh 2012). In this book I have contributed to such scholarship by examining the central role of stories and storytelling in that process.

The approach I have taken focuses on three key aspects of stories and their telling: emplotment, multimodal poetics, and circulation. These three aspects roughly correspond to Paul Ricoeur's (1984) discussion of three types of mimesis in narrative (46), or what has been described as the narrated event (what happens in the story), the narrative itself (the linguistic/poetic devices through which the story is told), and the narrative event (the social activity in which the story is told) (Bauman 1986: 2). Such an approach attends to stories in terms of not only their content but also their linguistic construction and social context.

The examination of emplotment, particularly the analysis of how grammatical tense and other markers of temporality are deployed in a story, provides information about how storytellers link past, present, and future. By linking distinct actions and events, especially those that are not spatially or temporally contiguous, stories make claims about causal relationships (Ochs 2004). Through emplotment, one can explain what one should have done, could do in the present, and should do in the future. One can also make epistemic claims about how one event or action is linked to another. In this way, emplotment is central to the constitution of values.

The examination of multimodal poetics provides information about how storytellers communicate affect, infusing their stories with emotion. In stories that feature visual and auditory aids (e.g., imagery, videos, music), multimodal poetics relies heavily on conventional existing emotion-laden interpretations of particular types of images and musical patterns. Though not explored in this book, poetics also offers connections within a narrative through parallel grammatical constructions (the repetition of a linguistic pattern accompanied by a change in focus). On a broader time-scale, though, the recontextualization of stories across speakers and sites discussed in this book is itself a kind of parallelism, where storytellers' management of the differences between their telling and others (the management of intertextual gaps—see Briggs and Bauman 1992) connects meaning-making in one storytelling event to another. Multimodal poetics is especially significant in the constitution of ethical values, where notions of causality and possibility meet understandings of good and bad, right and wrong.

Finally, the examination of circulation provides information about the social life of stories. Here, the case of contemporary global health storytelling is particularly instructive because of the socioeconomic organization of the field, relying as it does on philanthropy for a significant amount of its funding. Those who donate to an NPO become implicitly authorized to tell that NPO's story. Furthermore, even when donors avoid telling such stories, others may do so on their behalf, laminating social/ethical value onto the persona of the philanthropist. The circulation and transformation of stories in which values are constituted is a key way that those values themselves are circulated and transformed.

The weaving of plots—using multimodal poetic devices for particular audiences—is an imaginative act. At the same time, this creative process is heavily shaped by linguistic and communicative conventions, socioeconomic structures and histories, and the need to manage intertextual gaps to ensure that the story is comprehensible and interpretable by particular target audiences. Such conventionality narrows the wide scope of possibility to a vector of probability, a narrowing that thus occurs through the very same creative process of storytelling that allows possibilities to be imagined into being in the first place. It is through this push and pull that global health futures are imagined into being and thus can be transformed.

Notes

1 https://www.gatesfoundation.org/ideas/articles/childhood-mortality-south-africa-champs-soweto. Accessed 10/19/2023.
2 https://www.who.int/initiatives/action-on-the-social-determinants-of-health-for-advancing-equity/world-report-on-social-determinants-of-health-equity/commission-on-social-determinants-of-health#:~:text=The%20Commission%20on%20Social%20Determinants,ill%20health%20and%20health%20inequities. Accessed 10/19/2023.
3 https://www.cdc.gov/about/sdoh/index.html. Accessed 10/19/2023.
4 https://www.youtube.com/watch?v=4skQyHD8kRU&t=32s, https://www.youtube.com/watch?v=rJEk_RzqUAE, and https://www.youtube.com/watch?v=hWvDCGY86S0. Accessed 10/27/2023.
5 https://www.youtube.com/watch?v=E2q_VxS24sM. Accessed 10/27/2023.
6 https://www.gatesfoundation.org/ideas/media-center/press-releases/2011/11/foundation-announces-$35-million-in-funding-for-innovative-ideas-in-family-health. Accessed 10/27/2023.

References

Abramowitz, Sharon, Meredith Marten, and Catherine Panter-Brick. 2014. "Medical Humanitarianism: Anthropologists Speak Out on Policy and Practice." *Medical Anthropology Quarterly* 29 (1): 1–23.

Adams, Vincanne, ed. 2016. *Metrics: What Counts in Global Health*. Durham, NC: Duke University Press.

Alim, H. Samy, John R. Rickford, and Arnetha F. Ball, eds. 2016. *Raciolinguistics: How Language Shapes Our Ideas About Race*. New York: Oxford University Press.

Baker, Lee D. 2021. "The Racist Anti-Racism of American Anthropology." *Transforming Anthropology* 29 (2): 127–142.

Bauman, Richard. 1986. *Story, Performance, and Event: Contextual Studies of Oral Narrative*. New York: Cambridge University Press.

Blevins, John, Elizabeth O'Mara Sage, Ahoua Kone, Maria Maixenchs, Pratima L. Raghunathan, Rui A. Guilaze, Saquina Cossa, Zerihun Girma, Yosef Zegeye, Caroline Ackley, Faruque Hussain, Saiful Islam, Nellie Myburgh, Noni Ngwenya, Shabir A. Madhi, Petrer Otieno, Kennedy Ochola, Khátia Munguambe, and

Robert F. Breiman. 2019. "Using Participatory Workshops to Assess Alignment or Tension in the Community for Minimally Invasive Tissue Sampling Prior to the Start of Child Mortality Surveillance: Lessons from 5 Sites across the CHAMPS Network." *Clinical Infectious Diseases* 69: S280–S290.

Brada, Betsey Behr. 2011. "'Not *Here*': Making the Spaces and Subjects of 'Global Health' in Botswana." *Culture, Medicine, and Psychiatry* 35 (2): 285–312.

Brada, Betsey Behr. 2017. "Exemplary or Exceptional? The Production and Dismantling of Global Health in Botswana." In *Global Health and Geographical Imaginaries*, edited by Clare Herrick and David Reubi, 40–53. New York: Routledge.

Briggs, Charles L. 2024. "Incommunicable: Decolonizing Perspectives on Language and Health." *American Anthropologist* 126 (1): 83–95.

Briggs, Charles L., and Richard Bauman. 1992. "Genre, Intertextuality, and Social Power." *Journal of Linguistic Anthropology* 2 (2): 131–172.

Bucholtz, Mary, Dolores Inés Casillas, and Jin Sook Lee. 2016. "Beyond Empowerment: Accompaniment and Sociolinguistic Justice in a Youth Research Program." In *Sociolinguistic Research: Application and Impact*, edited by Robert Lawson and Dave Sayers, 25–44. New York: Routledge.

Darnell, Regna. 1998. *And Along Came Boas: Continuity and Revolution in Americanist Anthropology*. Philadelphia, PA: John Benjamins.

Fluehr-Lobban, Carolyn. 2000. "Anténor Firmin: Haitian Pioneer of Anthropology." *American Anthropologist* 102 (3): 449–466.

Graber, Kathryn E. 2023. "Textures of Value: Tactility, Experience, and Exclusion in the Cashmere Commodity Chain." *Economic Anthropology* 10 (2): 186–196.

Graeber, David. 2001. *Toward an Anthropological Theory of Value: the False Coin of Our Own Dreams*. New York: Palgrave.

Kerry, Vanessa, Agnes Binagwaho, Jonathan Weigel, and Paul Farmer. 2014. "From Aid to Accompaniment: Rules of the Road for Development Assistance." In *The Handbook of Global Health Policy*, edited by Garrett W. Brown, Gavin Yamey, and Sarah Wamala, 483–504. Malden, MA: Wiley.

Kockelman, Paul. 2016. *The Chicken and the Quetzal: Incommensurate Ontologies and Portable Values in Guatemala's Cloud Forest*. Durham, NC: Duke University Press.

Kockelman, Paul. 2020. *Kinds of Value: An Experiment in Modal Anthropology*. Chicago, IL: Prickly Paradigm Press.

Nguyen, Vinh-Kim. 2008. "Antiretroviral Globalism, Biopolitics, and Therapeutic Citizenship." In *Global Assemblages: Technology, Politics, and Ethics as Anthropological Problems*, edited by Aihwa Ong and Stephen J. Collier, 124–144. Oxford: Blackwell Publishing.

Ochs, Elinor. 2004. "Narrative Lessons." In *A Companion to Linguistic Anthropology*, edited by Alessandro Duranti, 269–289. Malden, MA: Blackwell Publishers.

Rabinow, Paul, and Nikolas Rose. 2006. "Biopower Today." *Biosocieties* 1 (2): 195–217.

Ricoeur, Paul. 1984. *Time and Narrative*. Chicago, IL: University of Chicago Press.

Rosa, Jonathan, and Vanessa Díaz. 2020. "Raciontologies: Rethinking Anthropological Accounts of Institutional Racism and Enactments of White Supremacy." *American Anthropologist* 122 (1): 120–132.

Shankar, Shalini, and Jillian R. Cavanaugh. 2012. "Language and Materiality in Global Capitalism." *Annual Review of Anthropology* 41: 355–369.

Volosinov, V. N. 1973 [1929]. *Marxism and the Philosophy of Language*. Translated by Ladislav Matejka and I. R. Titunik. Cambridge, MA: Harvard University Press.

Weigel, Jonathan, Matthew Basilico, and Paul Farmer. 2013. "Taking Stock of Foreign Aid." In *Reimagining Global Health: An Introduction*, edited by Paul Farmer, Arthur Kleinman, Jim Kim and Matthew Basilico, 287–301. Berkeley: University of California Press.

Yam, Eileen A., Martha Silva, Malini Ranganathan, Jamila White, Tonija M. Hope, and Chandra L. Ford. 2021. "Time to Take Critical Race Theory Seriously: Moving Beyond a Colour-Blind Gender Lens in Global Health." *The Lancet Global Health* 9 (4): E389–E390.

Yates-Doerr, Emily. 2020. "Reworking the Social Determinants of Health: Responding to Material-Semiotic Indeterminancy in Public Health Interventions." *Medical Anthropology Quarterly* 34 (3): 378–397.

Index

FSC www.fsc.org
MIX
Papier | Fördert gute Waldnutzung
FSC® C083411

Kolibri 360 GmbH
Ferdinand-Jühlke-Straße 7
99095 Erfurt, Deutschland
produktsicherheit@kolibri360.de